Oral Cancer

Editors

ERIC T. STOOPLER
THOMAS P. SOLLECITO

DENTAL CLINICS OF NORTH AMERICA

www.dental.theclinics.com

January 2018 • Volume 62 • Number 1

ELSEVIER

1600 John F. Kennedy Boulevard • Suite 1800 • Philadelphia, Pennsylvania, 19103-2899

http://www.dental.theclinics.com

DENTAL CLINICS OF NORTH AMERICA Volume 62, Number 1
January 2018 ISSN 0011-8532, ISBN: 978-0-323-58302-2

Editor: John Vassallo; j.vassallo@elsevier.com
Developmental Editor: Laura Fisher

Dental Clinics of North America (ISSN 0011-8532) is published quarterly by Elsevier Inc., 360 Park Avenue South, New York, NY 10010-1710. Months of issue are January, April, July, and October. Business and Editorial Offices: 1600 John F. Kennedy Boulevard, Suite 1800, Philadelphia, PA 19103-2899. Periodicals postage paid at New York, NY and additional mailing offices. Subscription prices are $294.00 per year (domestic individuals), $581.00 per year (domestic institutions), $100.00 per year (domestic students/residents), $364.00 per year (Canadian individuals), $751.00 per year (Canadian institutions), $422.00 per year (international individuals), $751.00 per year (international institutions), and $200.00 per year (international and Canadian students/residents). International air speed delivery is included in all *Clinics* subscription prices. All prices are subject to change without notice. **POSTMASTER:** Send address changes to *Dental Clinics of North America*, Elsevier Health Sciences Division, Subscription Customer Service, 3251 Riverport Lane, Maryland Heights, MO 63043. **Customer Service (orders, claims, online, change of address): Elsevier Health Sciences Division, Subscription Customer Service, 3251 Riverport Lane, Maryland Heights, MO 63043. Tel: 1-800-654-2452 (U.S. and Canada). Fax: 314-447-8029. E-mail: journalscustomer service-usa@elsevier.com (for print support); journalsonlinesupport-usa@elsevier.com (for online support).**

Reprints. For copies of 100 or more, of articles in this publication, please contact the Commercial Reprints Department, Elsevier Inc., 360 Park Avenue South, New York, NY 10010-1710. Tel.: 212-633-3874; Fax: 212-633-3820; E-mail: reprints@elsevier.com.

The Dental Clinics of North America is covered in *MEDLINE/PubMed (Index Medicus), Current Contents/Clinical Medicine, ISI/BIOMED* and *Clinahl.*

Contributors

EDITORS

ERIC T. STOOPLER, DMD, FDSRCS, FDSRCPS
Associate Professor of Oral Medicine, University of Pennsylvania School of Dental Medicine, Philadelphia, Pennsylvania, USA

THOMAS P. SOLLECITO, DMD, FDS RCSEd
Professor and Chairman of Oral Medicine, University of Pennsylvania School of Dental Medicine, Philadelphia, Pennsylvania, USA

AUTHORS

SUNDAY O. AKINTOYE, BDS, DDS, MS
Director of Oral Medicine Research Program, Associate Professor, Department of Oral Medicine, University of Pennsylvania School of Dental Medicine, Philadelphia, Pennsylvania, USA

FAIZAN ALAWI, DDS
Associate Professor, Department of Pathology, University of Pennsylvania School of Dental Medicine, Philadelphia, Pennsylvania, USA

ROXANNE BAVARIAN, DMD
Division of Oral Medicine and Dentistry, Brigham and Women's Hospital, Harvard School of Dental Medicine, Boston, Massachusetts, USA

ADITI BHATTACHARYA, BDS, MDS, PhD
Assistant Professor, Department of Oral and Maxillofacial Surgery, NYU College of Dentistry, New York, New York, USA

MICHAEL T. BRENNAN, DDS, MHS
Professor and Chair, Department of Oral Medicine, Carolinas HealthCare System, Carolinas Medical Center, Charlotte, North Carolina, USA

LEE HARTNER, MD
Clinical Associate Professor of Medicine, University of Pennsylvania, Abramson Cancer Center, Philadelphia, Pennsylvania, USA

MICHAELL A. HUBER, DDS
Professor, Department of Comprehensive Dentistry, UT Health San Antonio School of Dentistry, San Antonio, Texas, USA

ALEXANDER ROSS KERR, DDS, MSD
Clinical Professor, Department of Oral and Maxillofacial Pathology, Radiology and Medicine, NYU College of Dentistry, New York, New York, USA

RAJESH V. LALLA, DDS, PhD, DABOM
Associate Professor of Oral Medicine, Associate Dean for Research, UConn Health, Farmington, Connecticut, USA

LAUREN E. LEVI, DMD
Clinical Instructor, Department of Dentistry, Icahn School of Medicine at Mount Sinai, New York, New York, USA

CHIA-CHENG LI, DDS, DMSc
Instructor, Department of Oral Medicine, Infection and Immunity, Harvard School of Dental Medicine, Boston, Massachusetts, USA

ALEXANDER LIN, MD
Department of Radiation Oncology, Perelman School of Medicine University of Pennsylvania, Philadelphia, Pennsylvania, USA

MEL MUPPARAPU, DMD, MDS, Diplomate, ABOMR
Professor and Director of Radiology, Attending, Oral Medicine, Department of Oral and Maxillofacial Surgery, Hospital of the University of Pennsylvania, Philadelphia, Pennsylvania, USA

CHRISTINE NADEAU, DMD, MSc
Associate Professor, Oral Medicine, Program Director, Faculty of Dentistry, Université Laval, Québec, Québec, Canada

BERT W. O'MALLEY Jr, MD, FACS
Gabriel Tucker Professor and Chair, Department of Otorhinolaryngology/Head and Neck Surgery, Perelman School of Medicine University of Pennsylvania, Philadelphia, Pennsylvania, USA

RABIE M. SHANTI, DMD, MD
Assistant Professor of Oral and Maxillofacial Surgery and Pharmacology, University of Pennsylvania School of Dental Medicine, Assistant Professor of Otorhinolaryngology/ Head and Neck Surgery, Perelman School of Medicine University of Pennsylvania, Philadelphia, Pennsylvania, USA

ZHEN SHEN, PhD
Harvard School of Dental Medicine, Boston, Massachusetts, USA

TAKAKO IMAI TANAKA, DDS, FDS RCSEd
Professor, Department of Oral Medicine, University of Pennsylvania School of Dental Medicine, Philadelphia, Pennsylvania, USA

JESUS AMADEO VALDEZ, DDS, MAS
Resident, Department of Oral Medicine, Carolinas HealthCare System, Carolinas Medical Center, Charlotte, North Carolina, USA

ALESSANDRO VILLA, DDS, PhD, MPH
Instructor, Department of Oral Medicine, Infection, and Immunity, Harvard School of Dental Medicine, Associate Surgeon, Division of Oral Medicine and Dentistry, Brigham and Women's Hospital, Boston, Massachusetts, USA

FAN YANG, DDS, PhD
Harvard School of Dental Medicine, Boston, Massachusetts, USA

Contents

Evaluation and Management of Oral Potentially Malignant Disorders   1

Christine Nadeau and Alexander Ross Kerr

> Oral potentially malignant disorders (OPMDs) refer to epithelial lesions and conditions with an increased risk for malignant transformation; oral leukoplakia is the most commonly encountered. Overall, OPMDs have a low risk for malignant transformation, yet the challenge is the difficulty to reliably identify and predict which patients with OPMDs are at the highest risk for malignant transformation. Future research is needed to elucidate the molecular aspects of OPMDs, to improve current diagnostic strategies, leading to personalized management.

Oral Cancer: Genetics and the Role of Precision Medicine   29

Chia-Cheng Li, Zhen Shen, Roxanne Bavarian, Fan Yang, and Aditi Bhattacharya

> Oral squamous cell carcinoma (OSCC) is one of the leading cancers in the world. Patients with OSCC are managed with surgery and/or chemoradiation. Prognoses and survival rates are dismal, however, and have not improved for more than 20 years. Recently, the concept of precision medicine was introduced, and the introduction of targeted therapeutics demonstrated promising outcomes. This article reviews the current understanding of initiation, progression, and metastasis of OSCC from both genetic and epigenetic perspectives. In addition, the applications and integration of omics technologies in biomarker discovery and drug development for treating OSCC are reviewed.

Evaluation and Staging of Oral Cancer   47

Mel Mupparapu and Rabie M. Shanti

> Although the American Joint Committee on Cancer developed its first cancer-specific staging system in 1959, the TNM classification, as it has become known, has undergone many revisions mainly because of the advancements in both diagnosis and management of cancer. Although the basic purpose of the cancer staging system has remained fundamentally unchanged, the ease with which the cancer can be staged has evolved with newer methods. This article reviews cancer evaluation for staging, as well as the introduction of a new staging method effective as of 2018.

Adjunctive Diagnostic Techniques for Oral and Oropharyngeal Cancer Discovery   59

Michaell A. Huber

> The most important prognostic factor in predicting the outcome of oral and oropharyngeal cancer (OPC) is the stage at which it is diagnosed. Only 30% of patients are diagnosed with early-stage disease. The oral health

care provider performs an important role in early diagnosis of oral cancer. The conventional oral examination consists of a visual and tactile assessment of accessible oral and head and neck structures. Any suspicious or equivocal lesion should be reevaluated within 4 weeks. Evidence supporting the use of adjunctive devices to improve the ability to screen for and identify OPCs and oral premalignant lesions remains low.

Today, most head and neck cancer subsites, such as the larynx, hypopharynx, nasopharynx, and oropharynx, are treated with radiation therapy with or without chemotherapy as a primary treatment modality. Surgery is reserved for the salvage of recurrent tumors that occur within the head and neck in the absence of distant (ie, lung, liver) metastasis. However, unlike all other head and neck subsites, oral cancer should ideally be managed with primary surgery with the possibility of adjuvant radiation therapy with or without chemotherapy depending on the presence of certain high-risk pathologic features.

The use of chemotherapy, including immunotherapy, in oral squamous cell carcinoma has expanded considerably in the past several years. Its use mirrors that in the treatment of squamous cell carcinoma affecting other structures in the head and neck. This article summarizes the current evidence that guides the use of chemotherapy both in combination with radiation and as monotherapy for patients with advanced disease. It also addresses the expanding role of immunotherapy, particularly use of programmed cell death-ligand 1 inhibitors, in the treatment of advanced disease.

Radiotherapy is a key therapeutic modality used in the treatment of oral cavity and oropharyngeal cancers, whether as definitive treatment or postoperatively for those with high-risk factors after surgery. Although radiotherapy is a proven, effective treatment of cancer control, it can result in significant acute and late toxicities. Pretreatment patient education, supportive care, and posttreatment adherence to rehabilitative and preventive care can help mitigate toxicities. Advances in radiation delivery, such as through continued technological advances, or novel approaches to customizing radiation dose and volume, to maximize the therapeutic efficacy while minimizing side effects, are warranted.

Human papillomavirus–associated oropharyngeal squamous cell carcinoma (HPV-OPSCC) comprises approximately 25% of all head and neck cancers (head and neck squamous cell carcinoma, HNSCC). Epidemiologic studies have shown a dramatic increase of HPV-OPSCC in the past 2 decades, whereas tobacco-related HNSCC rates are decreasing worldwide. The distinctions between HPV-OPSCC and oral cavity cancers are now reflected in the most recent editions of the World Health Organization Classification of Tumors of the Head and Neck and the American Joint Committee on Cancer Staging Manual, respectively. This review describes the current understanding of the link between HPV infection and OPSCC.

Oral cancer therapy is associated with a multitude of head and neck sequelae that includes, but is not limited to, hyposalivation, increased risk for dental caries, osteoradionecrosis of the jaw, radiation fibrosis syndrome, mucositis, chemotherapy-induced neuropathy, dysgeusia, dysphagia, mucosal lesions, trismus, and infections. Preparing a comprehensive treatment plan for patients undergoing cancer therapy is essential to help minimize their risks for developing these oral and dental complications. In addition, dentists must take into account a patient's ongoing oncologic therapy for those patients who present to the dentist while concurrently receiving cancer treatment.

Oral cancer therapies are associated with orofacial complications that could result in dose-limiting cancer treatment and consequent suboptimal tumor control. Oral cancer treatment complications include oral mucositis, salivary gland hypofunction, odontogenic infections, pain, dermatitis, neurotoxicity, soft tissue fibrosis, trismus, osteoradionecrosis, and potential cancer recurrence. These complications significantly affect cancer survivorship, quality of life, and psychosocial status. Effective dental management of patients with oral cancer involves the coordination of care among several health care professionals before, during, and after cancer therapy. The goal is to minimize complications and establish optimal quality of life for survivors.

The clinical manifestations of oral cancer and the effects of treatment can have a negative impact on a patient's quality of life. Physiologic functions, cosmetic appearance, and psychological well-being can become compromised during the diagnosis, treatment, and survivorship of patients with oral cancer. This article addresses the relationship of oral cancer and quality of life, as well as the different aspects affected by this condition.

DENTAL CLINICS OF NORTH AMERICA

Preface
Oral Cancer

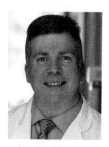 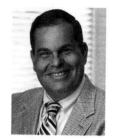

Eric T. Stoopler, DMD, FDSRCS, FDSRCPS   Thomas P. Sollecito, DMD, FDS RCSEd

Editors

This issue of *Dental Clinics of North America*, entitled *Oral Cancer*, is designed to update oral health care providers with clinically relevant information regarding this potentially devastating condition. Generally, there is decreased public awareness of oral cancer compared with other types of cancers, which are often less prevalent. Early detection of oral cancer is of critical importance as risk of metastatic disease increases and survival rates decrease with delayed diagnosis. Symptoms are often absent in the early stages of disease, which contributes to the difficulty of diagnosing this condition. In later stages, individuals with oral cancer can experience a range of signs and symptoms, including pain, loss of sensation, limited mouth opening, and/or difficulty swallowing. Clinically suspicious lesions for oral cancer are typically white and/or red in appearance and indurated on palpation. Tissue analysis of the lesion(s) is imperative to establish a definitive diagnosis. Comprehensive management of this condition often requires an interdisciplinary team of dental and medical professionals to address all aspects of patient care.

Oral health care providers are the primary vanguards against oral cancer. Identifying risk factors associated with oral cancer, such as use of tobacco, use of alcohol, and human papillomavirus infection, accompanied by relevant review of systems questions, should be incorporated into the medical history and subsequent updates at each patient visit. A conventional visual and tactile examination of the oral cavity and associated structures of the head and neck must be conducted for every patient and should be expected by patients at every dental appointment. Oral lesions exhibiting clinical signs and symptoms of frank malignancy or those clinically suspicious for potential malignancy should undergo biopsy. Innocuous lesions should be reevaluated in one month and may be subject to initial cytologic evaluation to determine the next appropriate course of action. Prompt referral to the appropriate dental and medical specialists should ensue if oral cancer is diagnosed for comprehensive patient evaluation and management.

Dent Clin N Am 62 (2018) ix–x
http://dx.doi.org/10.1016/j.cden.2017.09.002
0011-8532/18/© 2017 Published by Elsevier Inc.

dental.theclinics.com

True advancement in the detection and management of oral cancer will be based on basic science and clinical research. The important concept of personalized medicine in the context of human disease should be further explored and developed. Information about a patient's genes and/or cellular environment, utilizing sophisticated instruments to visualize biomarkers in tissue before clinical change is detected, and use of molecular-based cancer drugs to effectively target only tumor cells will be the most effective way to confront and eradicate oral cancer in the future.

All the contributing authors to this issue have been carefully selected and are renowned clinicians, educators, and researchers in their respective fields. It is our hope that the information contained herein will help enhance fundamental knowledge and clinical expertise as it relates to oral cancer with the goals of enhancing detection, optimizing management, and improving outcomes of patients with this condition.

DEDICATIONS

I dedicate this issue to my wife, Melanie, and my children, Ryan and Ethan, for their unconditional love, encouragement, and support of my professional endeavors. I also thank my parents, Francine and Stanley, for their love and guidance. I wish to acknowledge my mentors, colleagues, residents, students, and patients, who continually contribute to my professional development.

Eric T. Stoopler, DMD, FDSRCS, FDSRCPS

I dedicate this issue to my wife, Carolyn, and my children, Elizabeth, Peter, and Katharine, for their unconditional love and support of my academic pursuits. I also thank my parents, Clara and Peter, for their love and guidance. I wish to acknowledge my mentors, colleagues, residents, students, and patients, who continually contribute to my professional development.

Thomas P. Sollecito, DMD, FDS RCSEd

Eric T. Stoopler, DMD, FDSRCS, FDSRCPS
University of Pennsylvania
School of Dental Medicine
240 South 40th Street
Philadelphia, PA 19104, USA

Thomas P. Sollecito, DMD, FDS RCSEd
University of Pennsylvania
School of Dental Medicine
240 South 40th Street
Philadelphia, PA 19104, USA

E-mail address:
tps@upenn.edu

Evaluation and Management of Oral Potentially Malignant Disorders

CrossMark

Christine Nadeau, DMD, MSc[a],*, Alexander Ross Kerr, DDS, MSD[b]

KEYWORDS

- Oral potentially malignant disorders • Leukoplakia • Malignant transformation
- Risk assessment • Screening • Management

KEY POINTS

- Oral potentially malignant disorders (OPMDs) refer to epithelial lesions and conditions with an increased risk for malignant transformation; oral leukoplakia is the most commonly encountered.
- Overall, OPMDs have a low risk for malignant transformation, yet the challenge is the difficulty to reliably identify and predict which patients with OPMDs are at the highest risk for malignant transformation.
- Future research is needed to elucidate the molecular aspects of OPMDs, to improve current diagnostic strategies, leading to personalized management.

INTRODUCTION

Oral potentially malignant disorders (OMPDs) refer to all epithelial lesions and conditions with an increased risk for malignant transformation (MT).[1] OMPDs include different entities; oral leukoplakia (OL) is the most common OPMD[2] whereas oral erythroplakia (OE) is relatively uncommon (**Box 1**).[1,3] OL is defined as a "white plaque of questionable risk having excluded (other) known diseases or disorders that carry no increased risk for cancer."[2] It is a clinical diagnosis based on the history and examination findings and not based on specific histopathologic features. Clinically, OL is typically unifocal and presents as 2 clinical phenotypes: homogenous and nonhomogeneous. The homogeneous type typically appears as a flat, thin, uniform white plaque with or without fissuring[4] (**Fig. 1**). The nonhomogeneous type is nonuniform in appearance and may be subclassified into several different types, including

Disclosure Statement: No conflict.
[a] Faculty of Dentistry, Université Laval, Pavillon de Médecine dentaire, 2420 rue de la Terasse, Québec, Québec G1V 0A6, Canada; [b] Department of Oral and Maxillofacial Pathology, Radiology and Medicine, NYU College of Dentistry, 345 East 24th Street, New York, NY 10010, USA
* Corresponding author.
E-mail address: christine.nadeau@fmd.ulaval.ca

Dent Clin N Am 62 (2018) 1–27
http://dx.doi.org/10.1016/j.cden.2017.08.001
0011-8532/18/© 2017 Elsevier Inc. All rights reserved.

erythroleukoplakia a mixed red and white lesion but not predominantly white (**Fig. 2**), a speckled leukoplakia/leukoerythroplakia a mixed red and white lesion but predominantly white (**Fig. 3**), and nodular or verrucous leukoplakias (**Fig. 4**). In addition, OL may have a multifocal presentation, known as proliferative verrucous leukoplakia (PVL), which can have homogeneous and nonhomogenous features[1] (**Fig. 5**). OE is defined as "any lesion of the oral mucosa that presents as bright red velvety plaques which cannot be characterized clinically or pathologically as any other recognizable condition"[1,5] (**Fig. 6**).

Two other OPMDs that have a distinctly different pathogenesis compared with OL and OE include oral submucous fibrosis (OSMF) and oral lichen planus (OLP). OSMF is a chronic, insidious inflammatory disease stemming from areca nut chewing and characterized by a loss in fibroelasticity of the oral mucosa and submucosa.[6] OLP is a chronic inflammatory disease, characterized by a T lymphocyte–mediated immune response against epithelial basal cells, causing basal cell degeneration, which may result mucosal erosion and ulceration and commensurate oral soreness.[7] OPMDs may be exhibit epithelial dysplasia or, less frequently, oral squamous cell carcinoma

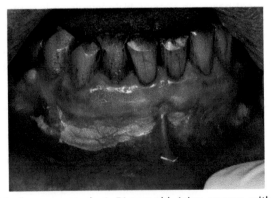

Fig. 1. Leukoplakia (homogeneous). A 51-year-old Asian woman with areca nut habit (paan). Note the extrinsic staining on teeth secondary to the habit. Definitive diagnosis was mild epithelial dysplasia.

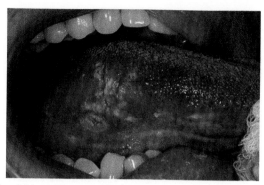

Fig. 2. Erythroleukoplakia. A 71-year-old white woman with a history of heavy alcohol use. Note the red and white colors of the lesion with ulcerated areas. The patient reported experiencing soreness and there was no induration on palpation. Definitive diagnosis was squamous cell carcinoma (T1N0M0).

(OSCC) at baseline presentation. Those that are not malignant are at risk for MT[1,8]; therefore, early detection and management of OMPDs are critical and may reduce the cancer-specific morbidity and mortality.[8,9] There is biopsychosocial morbidity associated with OPMDs, which can influence a patient's quality of life (QOL).[10] This article reviews the epidemiology, evaluation, and management of OPMDs, with an emphasis on OL, OE, PVL, OLP, and OSMF.

EPIDEMIOLOGY AND CLINICAL PRESENTATION

The worldwide reported prevalence of OPMDs (ie, number of cases identified in a given population at any one time) ranges from 1% to 5%.[11–13] This variable prevalence is dependent on the country of origin and lifestyle differences influencing the types of risk factors to which patients are exposed.[14,15] Similar to OSCC, OMPDs are predominantly associated with the use of tobacco, heavy alcohol consumption, and areca nut chewing,[16] although approximately 10% seem to have no known cause and are

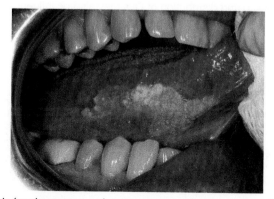

Fig. 3. Leukoplakia (nonhomogeneous). A 71-year-old white man with no history of tobacco use. Note an ulcerated area at the posterior aspect of the lesion and the thicker white area at the superior aspect of the lesion. Definitive diagnosis was moderate with focally severe epithelial dysplasia.

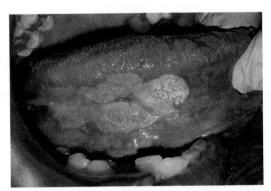

Fig. 4. Verrucous leukoplakia. A 74 -year-old white woman with no history of tobacco or alcohol use. Note the white lesion on the right lateral tongue harboring a verrucous appearing area. Definitive diagnosis was verrucous hyperplasia with mild epithelial dysplasia.

referred to as idiopathic.[14] The average age of patients with OPMDs is 50 years to 69 years,[17] and male-to-female ratio is approximately 3:1.[13,14] Incidence rates for OPMDs are largely based on data obtained from the Indian subcontinent (and therefore are biased), with a range between 0.6/1000 and 30.2/1000 (number of new cases per population at risk over a given time period).[18,19] OPMDs have a reported MT (MTR) of 0.13% to 36.4%[20] at an annual rate of 1.36% (95% CI, 0.69%–2.03%),[21] and the male-to-female MT ratio is approximately 1:2.[14]

Oral Leukoplakia

OL is the most common OPMD,[2,22] with an estimated worldwide prevalence of 2%[13] and with a predilection for men (male-to-female ratio of 3.22:1).[13] The prevalence is less than 1% in men under 30 years of age, whereas the prevalence rates in both men and women over the age of 70 are 8% and 2%, respectively.[17] It is seen 6 times more often among smokers than nonsmokers.[2] OL may affect any part of the oral cavity[23]; however, it most frequently involves the buccal mucosa (25%), gingiva (20%), and the floor of the mouth and ventrolateral tongue (10%), with the remainder dispersed among other sites (commissures, hard and soft palate, and alveolar ridges).[14] The oral site and distribution of OLs may also be influenced by the manner in which risk factors are used; for example, reverse cigar smoking causes lesions on the hard palate, and areca nut chewing predominantly causes buccal mucosal lesions

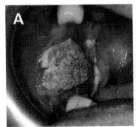
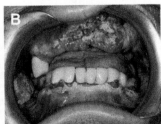
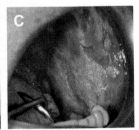

Fig. 5. PVL. A 68-year-old white woman with no history of tobacco or alcohol use. Note the multifocal white lesions on right buccal mucosa (A), maxillary and mandibular mucosa (B), and left buccal mucosa (C). Definitive diagnosis revealed 2 squamous cell carcinomas maxillary alveolar mucosa with bone invasion (T4aN0M0) and right buccal mucosa (T1N0M0).

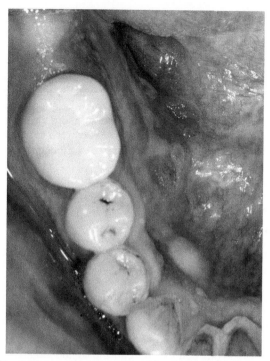

Fig. 6. Erythroplakia. A 56-year-old Asian man with a history of smoking and areca nut and heavy alcohol use. Definitive diagnosis was squamous cell carcinoma (T1N0M0).

at the site of placement.[24] The frequency of epithelial dysplasia in leukoplakia is approximately 1% to 30%.[25] Nonhomogenous OLs have a much higher chance of being dysplastic (12.63-fold) or demonstrating a focus of carcinoma (8.9-fold) compared with homogeneous OL.[26] The estimated overall MTR is 3.5% and typically occurs within the first 5 years.[16] A cross-sectional study in the United States reported the OL sites with the highest prevalence of severe dysplasia or carcinoma in situ were the floor of mouth (13.5%) and tongue (5%).[24,25]

Oral Erythroplakia

There is paucity of data on the epidemiology of OE and it is mostly based on retrospective analyses conducted in South Asia and Southeast Asia.[27] The prevalence ranges from 0.02% to 0.83%,[27] and OE predominantly affects the middle aged and elderly (sixth and seventh decades)[27] with no significant differences between genders.[28,29] The soft palate, floor of the mouth, and buccal mucosa are the most commonly affected sites (see **Fig. 5**). OE is usually asymptomatic, although patients may complain of a burning sensation associated with the lesion.[30] On biopsy and histopathologic evaluation, OE typically presents as severe epithelial dysplasia, carcinoma in situ, or microinvasive carcinoma. If not diagnosed as OSCC, it has the highest potential for MT among OPMDs with an MTR, ranging from 14% to 50%.[31] These data provide clinical relevance for biopsy site selection in an oral erythroleukoplakia because the red component of a mixed lesion is more likely to harbor the most severe pathology.[30]

Oral Lichen Planus

OLP affects 1% to 4% of the worldwide population of all races. Both genders may be affected with a higher frequency in women with 70% of affected women between the ages of 30 yearsto 60 years.[32] Clinically, OLP presents as different subtypes: a nonerosive-atrophic form (reticular, popular, and plaque-like) and an erosive-atrophic form (atrophic/erythematous, erosive/ulcerative, and bullous).[33] The most common site is the buccal mucosa, followed by the lateral tongue and gingiva.[34] The risk for MT of OLP is the subject of an ongoing and controversial discussion in the literature. A recent meta-analysis for risk of MT resulted in an overall pooled proportion of 1.1% (95% CI, 0.9%, 1.4%), with higher rates found among smokers (odds ratio [OR] 2; 95% CI, 1.25, 3.22), alcoholics (OR 3.52; 95% CI, 1.54, 8.03), and HCV infected patients (OR 5; 95% CI, 1.56, 16.07).[35] The most common type of OLP to undergo MT is the erosive form[35] and most common locations for MT are the tongue followed by buccal mucosa.[34]

Oral Submucous Fibrosis

OSMF is predominantly encountered in Southeast Asia, where the use of areca nut is most prevalent, but it may also be encountered in countries like the United Kingdom, the United states, and other developed countries with Southeast Asians immigrant populations.[36] OSMF is associated with the habitual chewing of areca nut preparations, most commonly as a betel quid or in single-use packets as pan masala or gutkha.[37] OSMF is mostly seen in young adults (ages 20–40) and affects the buccal mucosa, retromolar area, tongue, and soft palate.[37] Clinically, OSMF presents with progressive fibrosis of the oral soft tissues, causing limited mouth opening and diminished oral function, blanching of the oral mucosa, and a burning sensation (**Fig. 7**).[38] Fibrosis is irreversible, even after cessation of the chewing habit.[39] OSMF is associated with significant morbidity and mortality. Studies have reported the presence of dysplasia in approximately 25% of biopsied OSMF cases and the MTRs vary from 3% to 19%.[36,40] OSMF associated with OL is known to increase the risk for MT.[36]

Proliferative Verrucous Leukoplakia

This clinical entity was first described in 1985 by Hansen and colleagues.[41] PVL is characterized by multifocal lesions with a high risk for MT[42] (see **Fig. 4**). Patients with PVL have a mean age of 66.8 years and are mostly women, with a female-to-male ratio of 2.72:1.[43] It has a weak association with tobacco because it may occur

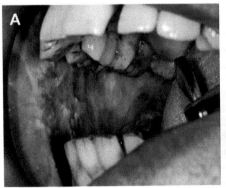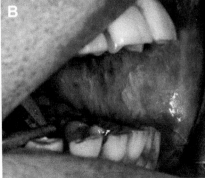

Fig. 7. OSMF. A 47-year-old Indian man with history of areca nut use. Note blanching of the (*A*) right and (*B*) left buccal mucosa and limited mouth opening due to OSMF.

in both smokers and nonsmokers.[20] The most affected sites are the gingiva, followed by buccal mucosa and alveolar ridges.[43] Initially, PVL may present as a unifocal, homogeneous white plaque and this creates difficulty in the early diagnosis of PVL given the overlapping clinical and histopathologic features of a homogeneous leukoplakia.[44] Early PVL lesions may also be mistaken for OLP (especially the reticular and plaque variants) because they may share certain subtle pathologic features (such as the presence of dense lichenoid chronic inflammation).[45] PVL gradually evolves to multifocal disease with a range of presentations, including white lesions, which often have a verrucous appearance, or mixed red and white lesions, some with ulceration. Over time, biopsy specimens show varying degrees of epithelial hyperplasia and dysplasia and eventually squamous carcinoma (verrucous or conventional squamous cell).[44] Diagnosis is based on a combination of these clinical and histopathologic features.[45] PVL's multifocal involvement makes it more difficult to manage surgically.[4] It is known for its high MTR (60%–100%), frequent recurrences after total excision (87%–100%), and high mortality rates (30%–50%).[46–48] The etiology of PVL is unknown; few studies have suggested possible etiologies related to lifestyle habits (tobacco use and alcohol use),[41,49] infectious agents (human papillomavirus, *Candida albicans*, and Epstein-Barr virus)[43] but none has demonstrated an association.

NATURAL HISTORY AND MALIGNANT TRANSFORMATION OF ORAL POTENTIALLY MALIGNANT DISORDERS

The natural history of an OPMD is variable, its evolution is not necessarily linear, and its propensity for progression to malignancy is difficult to predict. This creates challenges in the assessment and the management of OPMDs. Factors associated with an increased likelihood of MT are inherent to patients (age >45 years old, female gender, and nonsmoking status) and to clinical features such as anatomic sites (high risk sites include floor of the mouth, ventrolateral tongue, retromolar area, and soft palate),[16,50,51] size (lesions with size >200 mm^2 have shown a >5-fold increase in the risk of MT[51]), clinical phenotype (nonhomogeneous leukoplakia), and a higher grade of dysplasia.[16] Mehanna and colleagues[52] reported that OPMDs with high-grade dysplasia are more than twice as likely to undergo MT (mild/moderate 10.3% vs severe 24.1%). **Box 2** summarizes the risk factors for MT of OPMDs. A deeper understanding about the aberrant molecular pathways leading to carcinogenesis have led to the identification of potential markers that can help to predict which OPMDs are more likely to undergo MT. Loss of heterozygosity at key chromosomal loci (eg, 3p14, 9p21) and DNA ploidy are 2 examples of predictive biomarkers that have

---

Box 2
Risk factors for oral potentially malignant disorders malignant transformation

Female gender

Age greater than 45 years old

Leukoplakia in nonsmoker

Nonhomogeneous type

Size greater than 200 mm^2

Higher grade of dysplasia

High risk site (floor of mouth, ventrolateral tongue, retromolar area, soft palate)

been validated in longitudinal studies.[53,54] Other biomarkers are under investigation and are reviewed in Chia-Cheng Li and colleagues' article, "Oral Cancer: Genetics and the Role of Precision Medicine," in this issue.

EVALUATION
Screening

Screening for and the early detection of both OPMDs and OSCC can reduce the cancer-specific morbidity and mortality.[8,9] A recent review by the Global Oral Cancer Forum[55] reported that there was insufficient research evidence that population screening (ie, a national screening program) reduces mortality from oral cancer. The main issues were the relative rarity of the disease, the lack of knowledge of the natural history of the disease, and the lack of evidence on the efficacy and cost-effectiveness of different screening methods.[55] Lack of evidence regarding the benefits and harms of screening for oral cancer in asymptomatic adults in primary care settings was also reported by the United States Preventive Service Task Force.[56] Opportunistic screening for OPMDs and oral cancer during dental visits are recommended by the American Dental Association, Canadian Dental Association, and American Academy of Oral Medicine.[57] Oral cancer screening is not an isolated event but rather 1 component of the comprehensive head and neck examination[58] and represents an opportunity to assess any oral abnormalities, whether neoplastic, infectious, reactive/inflammatory, or developmental.[58] Such opportunistic screenings should be performed not only during a new patient examination but also at recalls and emergency or problem-focused visits for all patients,[59] particularly in those who use tobacco or who consume alcohol heavily.[58] **Fig. 8** summarizes a possible clinical algorithm for opportunistic screening of mucosal abnormalities including OPMDs.

Comprehensive Head and Neck Evaluation

A patient's evaluation must include the collection of demographic data; a detailed health history, including a patient's chief complaint; and medical, social, and dental histories. OPMDs are often asymptomatic, although if a patient presents with a chief complaint (ie, pain), it is important to record all details about the onset and clinical course. Risk assessment for OPMDs should specifically include details related to medical conditions associated with immunosuppression, a past history of cancer (or family history of cancer), habits (tobacco, alcohol, and areca nut use), poor diet or nutritional deficiencies, and any environmental exposures. A comprehensive head and neck examination consists of a visual and tactile examination. This begins with an extraoral examination to detect any head and neck asymmetry and skin lesions and includes palpation of midline neck structures (such as the thyroid gland), lymph nodes, and major salivary glands. Adults with persistent neck lymphadenopathy with no apparent explanation should be evaluated to rule out malignancy[60] and should trigger a careful intraoral examination to detect a primary OSCC if present (**Fig. 9**). In the absence of an obvious primary cancer, patients must be referred for further evaluation (ie, imaging or a fine-needle aspiration of the involved node[s]). Signs suggestive of neurologic dysfunction may include paresthesia/dysesthesia or loss of function indicating possible nerve invasion, and this warrants a complete cranial nerve examination. The intraoral examination must include inspection and palpation of all mucosal surfaces, and the visual detection of mucosal abnormalities warrants careful evaluation of the clinical features (such as location, morphology, color, and size). Palpation of a lesion revealing firmness/induration or pain is an ominous feature. High-risk sites

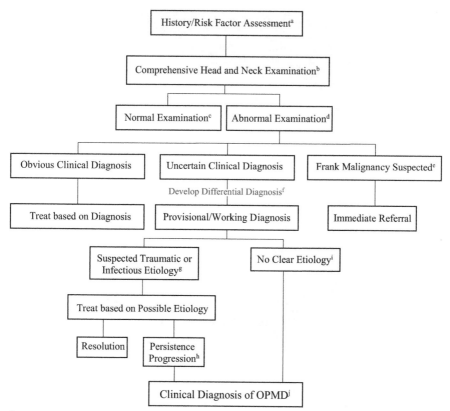

Fig. 8. Opportunistic screening for mucosal abnormalities including OPMDs. [a] History/risk factor assessment: include patient's chief complaint, medical/dental/social history, demographic data, and review of systems. Risk assessment specific for OPMDs includes medical conditions associated with immunosuppression, past history or family history of cancer, habits (tobacco, alcohol, and areca nut), poor diet/nutritional deficiencies, and environmental exposure. [b] Comprehensive head and neck examination: extraoral examination (visual and tactile examination to detect any abnormalities: head and neck asymmetry, skin lesion, palpation of midline and lateral structures, lymph nodes and major salivary glands, and cranial nerve examination). Intraoral examination (inspection and palpation of all mucosal surfaces. High risk sites: floor of mouth, ventrolateral border of the tongue, retromolar area, and soft palate). [c] Normal examination: findings are normal or within normal limits. [d] Abnormal examination: Document clinical features, such as morphology, location, color, size, and palpation of lesion revealing firmness/induration or pain. [e] Frank suspected malignancy: should be immediately referred for definitive diagnosis and management. [f] Develop a differential diagnosis: with provisional/working diagnosis at the top, initiate a diagnostic process to establish the definitive diagnosis. [g] Suspected traumatic or infectious etiology: remove all sources of mechanical, thermal or chemical irritation, treat infectious etiology. Reassess in 3 weeks to 4 weeks to confirm resolution or persistence/progression. [h] Persistence/progression: having eliminated possible etiology, if the lesion is persistent or progressive a clinical diagnosis of an OPMD is made. [i] No clear etiology: a clinical diagnosis of an OPMD is made when the clinician cannot identify the lesion or condition as otherwise benign based on the available history and physical findings. [j] Clinical diagnosis of OPMD: see **Fig. 10** for potential management strategies for patients with OPMDs.

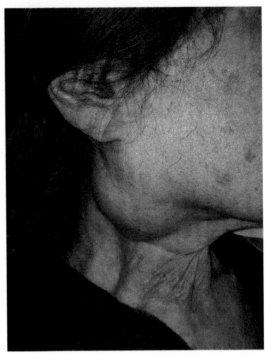

Fig. 9. Persistent lymphadenopathy. A 69-year-old white woman with a fixed firm non-tender right lymphadenopathy secondary metastasis from a recurrent SCC of the left lateral tongue (the lymph drainage was directed contralaterally due to a previous history of a selective neck dissection and adjuvant radiation treatment to the left side).

include the floor of mouth, ventrolateral tongue, retromolar area, and palate. Digital photographs provide an excellent way to record any abnormalities and may be useful to serially monitor mucosal abnormality progression.

The clinical diagnosis of an OPMD, such as an OL, is made when a clinician cannot identify the lesion or condition as otherwise benign based on the available history and physical findings. Clinicians should always develop a differential diagnosis when the clinical diagnosis is uncertain. This is a list of 2 or more clinical diagnoses ordered with the most likely, known as the working diagnosis, on top. This process initiates a diagnostic process to establish the definitive diagnosis. As an example, **Box 3** lists different benign clinical diagnoses that might be considered in a differential diagnosis for oral white lesions. These diagnoses must be considered or ruled out before a working diagnosis of an OPMD is made. The most common clinical diagnosis for a persistent white lesion is a frictional keratosis. If a clinician suspects a traumatic etiology, then the frictional keratosis is the working diagnosis, and leukoplakia may be considered as part of the differential. An attempt must be made to remove the source of mechanical, thermal, or chemical irritation and to reassess the patient in 3 weeks to 4 weeks to confirm the lesion is resolving. If a lesion persists and/or demonstrates evidence of progression, a clinical diagnosis of an OPMD is made and becomes the main working diagnosis. In all cases, a clinical diagnosis of an OPMD mandates biopsy to establish the definitive diagnosis and rule out dysplasia or OSCC. Depending on the clinician's training and experience, prompt referral of patients with OPMDs to a

---

Box 3
White lesions of the oral cavity

Reactive/frictional
  Leukoedema
  Linea alba
  Mordicatio
  White hairy tongue
  Frictional keratosis
  Smokeless tobacco keratosis
  Nicotinic stomatitis

Infectious
  Pseudomembranous candidiasis
  Hyperplastic candidiasis
  Human papilloma virus infection
  Hairy leukoplakia associated with Epstein-Barr virus

Immune mediated/autoimmune
  OLP
  Lichenoid reaction
  Benign migratory glossitis
  Systemic lupus erythematosus
  Discoid lupus erythematosus
  Graft-versus-host disease

Developmental
  White sponge nevus

OPMDs/malignacy
  OL
  PVL
  OSMF
  OSCC

---

clinician with advanced training in the diagnosis and management of oral mucosal diseases, such as an oral medicine specialist, is recommended. Patients presenting with an OPMD with a high index of suspicion for malignancy (ie, a large mass, lymphadenopathy, or other ominous signs) should be immediately referred to a head and neck oncology team. At all times, patients should be informed of all findings, proposed evaluation, and management. Clinicians must be certain of patient comprehension and understanding, obtain informed consent, and document all relevant information in patient records.

Impact on Quality of Life

The biopsychosocial morbidity associated with OSCC has been established; however, there is paucity of literature on the QOL specific to patients with OPMDs.[61] Recently, Tadakamadla and colleagues[62] developed an OPMD QOL questionnaire to evaluate the subjective perceptions of the impact of OPMDs in 150 patients with OPMDs (n = 50 each for OL, OSMF, or OLP with age-matched and gender-matched controls). The study reported poorer QOL in OPMDs patients compared with controls and identified 4 main issues: (1) perceived lack of knowledge by health care professionals about OPMDs and the diagnostic process, with most patients reporting traumatic experiences (ie, multiple visits to multiple health care providers, and different kind of treatments, often with no relief); (2) the experience of physical impairment and functional limitations (ie, burning sensation while eating or performing oral hygiene, or limited mouth opening affecting mastication); (3) the reduction in psychological and social well-being, notably the fear of MT, and the frustration related to the chronic nature of the condition, with no specific treatment; and (4) the effects of treatment on daily life (financial impact, difficulty in keeping appointments, treatment satisfaction, and impact of risk factor modification/habit cessation, such as tobacco smoking). A weakness of the study included the heterogeneity of the population: OLP and OSMF patients are different populations in terms of QOL, especially for the physical impairment and functional limitations (the most important issue for patients) compared with OL/OE, which are typically asymptomatic. Nevertheless, patients' perceptions and the impact of OPMD diagnosis on a patient's QOL can have an impact on psychological and social well-being and should be part of the comprehensive evaluation process.

DIAGNOSIS OF ORAL POTENTIALLY MALIGNANT DISORDERS

The current gold standard for the definitive diagnosis of OPMDs is based on biopsy and histopathologic examination.[1,4] OPMDs may exhibit hyperplasia, hyperkeratosis, varying degrees of dysplasia, carcinoma in situ, or OSCC.[4] The diagnosis and grading of oral epithelial dysplasia are based on a combination of architectural and cytologic changes using a 3-tiered grading classification: mild, moderate, and severe, with severe dysplasia and carcinoma in situ considered synonymous (2005 World Health Organization Classification [**Table 1**]).[63] There can be considerable interobserver and intraobserver variations in the grading of dysplasia[64,65]; yet, despite these shortcomings histopathology remains the most important factor dictating management[4,66] (see **Fig. 8**).

Diagnostic adjunctive techniques for OPMDs and OSCC are commercially available to clinicians. Their clinical application may facilitate biopsy site selection (see **Fig. 2**) to identify the most severe pathology in patients with OPMDs harboring variable histology or for the surveillance of patients with OPMDs or history of oral cancer.[67] Diagnostic adjunctive techniques includes optical devices, vital staining, cytopathologic platforms, and salivary diagnostics.[68–70] The role of current and emerging diagnostic adjunctive techniques is reviewed in Michaell A. Huber's article, "Adjunctive Diagnostic Techniques for Oral Cancer Discovery," in this issue.

Table 1 Grading systems of oral epithelial dysplasia	
Grading	**Histopathologic Characteristics**
Mild dysplasia	The architectural disturbance is limited to the lower third of the epithelium accompanied by cytologic atypia.
Moderate dysplasia	The architectural disturbance extends into the middle third of the epithelium; however, architectural disturbance extending into the middle third of the epithelium with sufficient cytologic atypia is upgraded from moderate to severe dysplasia.
Severe dysplasia	The architectural disturbance involves greater than two-thirds of the epithelium showing architectural disturbance with associated cytologic atypia.
Carcinoma in situ	Full-thickness or almost full-thickness architectural disturbance in the viable cell layers accompanied by pronounced cytologic atypia.

Data from Barnes L, Eveson J, Reichart P, et al. World health organizations classification of tumour. In: Pathology & genetics of head and neck tumours. IARC Press, editor. Lyon (France): IARC Press; 2005. p. 177–8.

MANAGEMENT OF ORAL POTENTIALLY MALIGNANT DISORDERS
Introduction

As stated previously, overall, OPMDs have a low risk for MT, estimated to be a rate of approximately 1.36% per year.[13] As such, it is difficult to justify interventions that are unnecessarily aggressive or associated with potential adverse effects. Risk stratification of patients with OPMDs seem to be the key to selecting an appropriate management plan, each patient receiving treatment commensurate with the degree of risk for progression and MT. Currently, the factors used to stratify risk in OL/OE include clinical factors (eg, nonsmoking status, high-risk subsite, nonhomogeneous appearance, and size of lesion >200 mm) coupled with higher histologic grade.[16] Yet, such factors are imperfect and with the advent of genomics, proteomics, and metabolomics, it is the dawn of personalized medicine and the potential to identify biomarkers present in patients with OPMDs that are predictive for progression and MT, the possibility to translate this into a personalized intervention may become a reality.

A wide range of treatments has been advocated for OPMDs, ranging from habit/risk factor control to medical and surgical interventions, surveillance/close monitoring, and a combination of these strategies. It is critical to understand the rationale, indications, and evidence for both the efficacy and safety of these modalities/strategies in the management of OPMDs. Clinicians must be able to interpret the available scientific literature, and an important question to ask is which endpoint or endpoints should be measured to assess the efficacy of an intervention. The worst possible outcome of not treating OPMDs is a worsening of disease; therefore, interventions that can prevent progression and MT of OPMDs should provide the most meaningful benefit to patients. Multicenter randomized placebo-controlled studies with long-term follow-up (>5 years), using the MTR as the primary endpoint or, as previously stated, surrogate biomarkers that are predictive for MT are considered the gold standard for assessing efficacy. Unfortunately, there is a paucity of such studies because they require larger populations and are expensive to undertake, and only a few have used surrogate biomarkers. As such, most of the published studies assess clinical, histologic, or molecular (ie, using various biomarkers) endpoints that correlate with a resolution of OPMDs and, therefore, are amenable to shorter follow-up intervals. In addition to efficacy, the safety profile and the cost-effectiveness for these interventions are important. Current strategies for the management of OPMDs are summarized, limitations of reported interventions highlighted, and future research priorities recommended. The focus is on OL/OE and PVL. The management of OSMF and OLP is not specifically covered in this article, and readers are directed to excellent reviews.[71,72]

Habit Cessation

There are no specific prospective clinical RCTs with the primary aim of assessing the efficacy of habit cessation as an intervention for patients with OPMDs. There are data, however, from epidemiologic studies to show that a high percentage of OPMDs in tobacco users resolve after tobacco cessation. Roosaar and colleagues[73] followed a cohort of patients with OL in Sweden over 2 decades and showed that there was a statistically significant resolution of OL in patients who had quit smoking compared with those that had not quit. Gupta and colleagues[74] explored the effect of exposing patients to an annual tobacco cessation program on the presence of oral lesions in a large Indian cohort of tobacco users (n = 12,212) over a 10-year period and showed a substantial decrease in the incidence of OL. Martin and colleagues[75] showed a regression of OLs over a 6-week period after tobacco cessation in a military population of smokeless tobacco users, although these OLs were likely reactive lesions rather than true OPMDs. None of these 3 studies explored histopathologic outcomes nor did they use MT as an endpoint. Roed-Petersen and colleagues[76] similarly reported an almost 30% disappearance of OLs after 3 months of abstinence. Nevertheless, these studies suggest that there is a subset of white lesions in tobacco users (smoked or smokeless), classified as OPMDs, which do resolve after tobacco cessation. Vladimirov and colleagues[77] explored the effect of tobacco cessation on a cohort of patients with OPMDs who had undergone surgical excision, demonstrating that the patients who continued to smoke were significantly more likely to undergo an "unfavourable outcome" (ie, recurrence of the OPMD or MT). There are no similar studies exploring the effects of cessation of alcohol or areca nut use on resolution of OPMDs. In summary, these studies collectively support that it is prudent to strongly encourage cessation as a first-line intervention for patients with OPMDs who use tobacco.

Yet, the compelling and irrefutable evidence that tobacco, heavy alcohol intake, and areca nut use are established independent causative agents for OSCC and OPMDs abrogates the need for habit interventional studies and provides ample justification to integrate evidenced-based guidelines for tobacco[78] and alcohol cessation[79] into clinical practice. There are currently no established evidence-based guidelines for areca nut use cessation.

Medical Interventions

Chemoprevention is defined as the use of drugs, vitamins, or other agents to try to reduce the risk of, or delay the development or recurrence of, cancer. The rationale is to use agents that can modulate carcinogenesis. Many topical and systemic chemopreventive agents have been studied on OPMDs, albeit few rigorous trials have been conducted. A recent systematic Cochrane review published in 2016 identified 15 placebo-controlled chemopreventive RCTs for OPMDs.[80] These and other trials more recently published are summarized in **Table 2**, which provides a listing of the agents, their formulation, rationale for use, and their efficacy based on primary endpoints.

Malignant transformation as an endpoint

Only 2 RCTs, assessing 3 systemic agents (vitamin A [retinyl acetate], β-carotene, and a β-carotene/vitamin C combination), explored MT as an endpoint.[81,82] These studies did not reveal a significant reduction in MT between those receiving the active treatments versus placebo, and the small sample size and suboptimal follow-up make it is difficult to interpret these results. MT in the active treatment groups occurred more frequently after the discontinuation of the agents, and long-term efficacy has not been studied in patients receiving extended courses of these or other agents (ie, beyond 3 years).

Clinical resolution as an endpoint

Only 2 RCTs (assessing 3 systemic agents) demonstrated a statistically significant improvement in clinical resolution of OPMDs (defined as complete clinical resolution [CR]) compared with controls, namely vitamin A[81,83] (which also prevented the development of OPMDs at new sites), β-carotene,[81] and lycopene.[84] Topical bleomycin showed a positive but not statistically significant effect.[85] Many of the agents studied demonstrated partial lesion responses, although the clinical ramifications of a partial response are difficult to interpret. A significant proportion of patients who demonstrated complete or partial responses relapsed after the discontinuation of many of these agents.

Table 2
Medical interventions with randomized placebo-controlled studies

Agent	Rationale	Formulations	Trial (Endpoint)
Retinoids	Inhibiting growth and inducing cell differentiation	Systemic: 13-cis-retinoic acid[86]	+(HR)
		Topical: 0.1% 13-cis-retinoic acid gel 3×/d × 4 mo[115]	−
Vitamin A	Inhibiting growth and inducing cell differentiation	Vitamin A 200,000 IU po/wk × 6 mo[83]	+(CR), +(HR)
		Vitamin A 300,000 IU po/wk × 12 mo[81]	+(CR)
Carotenoids	Antioxidants/ scavenge free reactive oxygen species	β-carotene 10 mg/vitamin C 500 mg po daily × 12 mo[82]	−
		β-carotene 360 mg/wk po × 12 mo[81]	+(CR)
		Lycopene 4–8 mg/d po × 3 mo[84]	+(CR), +(HR)
Green tea extracts	Antioxidants due to tea polyphenols (ie EGCG)	Green tea capsules 3g 4×/d plus extract applied to lesions 3×/d × 6 mo[87]	−
		Green tea extracts 500, 750, 100 mg/m² po tid × 3 mo[116]	
Black raspberry	Antioxidants due to high anthocyanin content	Topical: black raspberry bioadhesive gel daily × 3 mo[88]	−
Chinese herbs	Anti-inflammatory	Zengshengping 4 tablets po tid × 8–12 mo[117]	−
Bowman-Birk inhibitor	Protease inhibitor vs carcinogenesis-associated proteolysis	Topical: Bowman-Birk inhibitor concentrate mouthwash swished bid × 6 mo[118]	−
Nonsteroidal anti-inflammatory drugs	Cyclooxygenase inhibition	Topical: 0.1% ketorolac rinse once/d × 3 mo[119]	−
		Celecoxib 100, 200, or 400 mg po bid × 3 mo[120]	
Bleomycin	Chemotherapy	Bleomycin in DMSO (1%) application once daily × 14 d[85]	−
Erlotinib	Epidermal growth factor receptor inhibition	Erlotinib 150 mg/d po × 12 mo[89]	−

Abbreviations: +, positive trial; −, negative trial; CR, complete remission; DSMO, dimethyl sulfoxide; EGCG, epigallocatechin gallate; HR, histologic remission.

Histopathologic improvement as an endpoint

Only 2 RCTs demonstrated a statistically significant improvement in histology of OPMDs compared with controls: 1 assessing 13-cis-retinoic acid[86] and the other lycopene.[84] Topical bleomycin showed a positive but not statistically significant effect.[85] There are no data about changes in histopathology after discontinuation of use.

Use of predictive biomarkers

Some studies assessed biomarkers that have been established as predictive for MT. Stich and colleagues[83] performed a Feulgen staining on tissue samples before and after the course of vitamin A, and performed a crude ploidy analysis, showing a reversal in the condensed chromatin. Li and colleagues[87] demonstrated a similar reduction in micronuclei from exfoliated cells in the active treatment group receiving green tea extracts. The black raspberry extract and erlotinib trials tested biopsied tissue for loss of heterozygosity and showed a significant reduction in for loss of heterozygosity in the active arms versus controls.[88,89] There are no data about changes in predictive biomarkers after discontinuation of use.

Safety

Serious adverse events were rare, and judging by the similar subject dropout rates between placebo and active treatment groups, most subjects tolerated the agents. The systemic retinoids trial led to predictable and dose-related cutaneous adverse events (ie, cheilitis, facial erythema, and peeling of the skin), and hypertriglyceridemia. Two subjects experienced conjunctivitis and hypertriglyceridemia, necessitating discontinuation.[86] Long-term β-carotene use has been linked to an increased risk for lung cancer in smokers.[90]

Quality of the studies reported

Overall, the RCTs for the medical interventions for OPMDs are deemed of poor quality, with significant bias.[80] For studies exploring similar agents, the pooling the data was impossible due to the high degree of heterogeneity.

Surgical Removal/Ablative Interventions

Surgical excision is the first-line modality for the treatment of oral cavity squamous cell carcinoma and is also the most common intervention for dysplastic OPMDs. The rationale is that by removing the lesion(s), the risk for MT is reduced. Yet, surgical excision does not take into consideration the concept that not all patients presenting with OPMDs harbor disease that is specifically localized to a discrete lesion with clinically evident margins that are commensurate with histologic and molecular disease-free margins. Margins can be indistinct, extending locally beyond the visible lesion or, in some cases, widespread involving multiple mucosal sites. The concept of "field cancerization" was introduced by Slaughter and colleagues[91] more than 60 years ago and further elucidated in the molecular era.[92] PVL exemplifies this "field effect" and as discussed previously, PVL patients have multifocal OPMDs with a high propensity for MT, irrespective of the surgical management of the OPMDs.[93] Field effects and disease-involved margins are important factors predicting local recurrence and MT after surgical excision, not only of oral cancer but also for OPMDs. The standard of care for OSSC excision is to take 0.5-cm to 1-cm wide margins with intraoperative (frozen sections) and postoperative histopathologic margin assessment. Given the low overall risk for MT of OPMDs, however, it is difficult to uniformly justify similarly aggressive oncologic excision, opting instead for 1-mm to 2-mm surgical margins with marginal assessment not uniformly performed. The creation of a wound in patients with incompletely excised lesions (ie, involved margins) might lead to an increased risk for proliferation of neoplastic clones (ie, that harbor significant genetic and epigenetic alterations) during the healing process, thereby promoting disease progression and is a subject of further discussion and investigation.[94]

There are no RCTs assessing surgical removal/ablative interventions, and the current evidence is comprised of both prospective and retrospective cross-sectional or observational cohort studies testing either a single modality or a comparison of 2 or more surgical modalities. The primary endpoints typically include remission rates (complete or partial remission), recurrence rates, and if there are sufficient follow-up data, some studies have rMTRs. Secondary measures after surgical treatments may include intraoperative and postoperative parameters (eg, bleeding, pain, swelling, healing time, and postoperative fibrosis), and safety issues. Unfortunately, the analysis of cost-effectiveness has not been addressed in the literature. The studies are heterogeneous in terms of sample size (many are small), the blend of OPMDs (often there is a low percentage of dysplastic OPMDs or the population lacks a representative spectrum of histopathology), and the follow-up (most of which are <5 years). The spectrum of surgical and ablative interventions, including traditional surgical excision, lasers, cryotherapy, and photodynamic therapy (PDT), is discussed.

Traditional surgical excision

Traditional surgical excision includes cold blade scalpel excision or electrocautery excision. A large systematic review conducted by Mehanna and colleagues[52] included 14 studies, and the meta-analysis demonstrated a significantly reduced MT rate in patients with dysplastic OPMDs who underwent traditional surgical excision compared with those who did not (5.4% vs 14.6%) and concluded that surgical excision seems to decrease but does not eliminate the risk of MT. Many of the studies included in the review were poor-quality cross-sectional and observational cohort studies and showed significant heterogeneity. Not included in the review by Mehanna and colleagues was a large retrospective study conducted by Arduino and colleagues[95] over a 16-year period in 207 patients with dysplastic OPMDs (135 mild-grade, 50 moderate-grade, and 22 severe-grade dysplasia). The investigators reported no statistical difference in MTRs in those who underwent surgical excision compared with those who did not.

Lasers

Despite the purchasing costs, lasers have largely supplanted traditional surgical excision to become the workhorse surgical modality in the management of OPMDs. Lasers may be used for excision (ie, using the laser to excise a lesion followed by histopathologic submission) or vaporization of the lesion. The CO_2 laser is the most frequently studied, and the justifications for use seem to be based on a reduced propensity for pain, reduced postoperative edema, improved hemostasis, and reduced scarring.[96,97] Similarly, the erbium–yttrium-aluminum-garnet laser has demonstrated reduced pain levels compared with conventional surgical excision.[98]

A recent review of the CO_2 laser used on OPMDs was conducted by Modegas-Vegara and colleagues[99] and included 17 studies reporting recurrence rates and MTRs of 3% to 41% and 0% to 15%, respectively, and a follow-up range of 1 year to 5 years. Due to heterogeneity of methodology and study results, pooled data were not available to identify factors predicting recurrence or MT. Individual studies using multivariate analyses, however, did report such predictive factors. Thomson and colleagues,[100] in a cohort of 590 patients, showed that lesion appearance (OE > OL), grade of dysplasia (ie, severe > mild), and the presence of a lichenoid infiltrate (no > yes) were predictive for disease-free survival (ie, no evidence of recurrence of OPMD). Other studies demonstrated higher rates of recurrence in patients with multifocal lesions,[101] in those who continued to smoke,[101] in those with a history of alcohol use,[102] and in those with a previous history of malignancy (oral or other types of cancer)[102] or where there was poor accessibility of the lesion margins.[103] None of the studies showed factors predicting MT, likely due to insufficient sample size and/or inadequate follow-up.

Cryotherapy

Observational studies have explored the efficacy of cryotherapy to treat OPMDs, all using clinical remission and recurrence rates as endpoints and reviewed by Yu and colleagues.[104] Liquid nitrogen may be applied by cotton pellet or using a topical spray (open-system), or the freezing may be applied by a probe (closed-system). Closed systems provided the most efficient delivery and typically led to complete clinical remission of OLs with 1 to 6 treatments. Few of the studies included long-term follow-up; a recurrence rate, of 24%, was reported in only 1 study[105]; and none of the studies assessed MT.

Photodynamic therapy

PDT is based on the generation of cytotoxic free radicals from the activation of a photosensitizer by an appropriate wavelength of light. The photosensitizer (eg, 5-aminolevulinic acid, which is converted to protoporphyrin IX), may be administrated topically, intralesionally, or systemically, allowing time for it to be accumulated in the target tissues. The affected tissues are then exposed to the light source (eg, a 635-nm red light delivered by a laser) leading to a reaction releasing reactive oxygen species and causing the cytotoxic effect.[106] The clinical trials assessing the efficacy of PDT to treat OPMDs have been systematically reviewed.[107,108] In the 16 PDT studies reported in the literature, 14 used topical PDT, and 4 used PDT with intralesional and systemic photosensitizers (2 studies used 2 treatment arms comparing topical and systemic delivery). Complete response rates ranged from 23% to 100% and recurrence rates from 0% to 36%, but only a few of the studies followed patients for more than 5 years. Jerjes and colleagues[109] conducted a prospective topical PDT study on the largest and best-characterized cohort of 147 dysplastic OPMDs with a mean follow-up of more than 7 years. The complete response rate was 81% and correlated with grade of dysplasia (ie, complete remission 100%, 82%, 81%, and 69% for mild, moderate, severe, and carcinoma in situ, respectively). The recurrence rate was 11.6%, and an MT was noted in 7.5% of the patients. Residual photosensitization is a major adverse effect when the photosensitizer is delivered systemically; however, the adverse effects of systemically delivered PDT are minimal and do include postoperative pain and swelling.

Surveillance (observation)

Surveillance of patients with OPMDs means periodic follow-up at specified time intervals. There are no established evidence-based guidelines for surveillance of patients with OPMDs; however, given that the risk for MT cannot be predicted, irrespective of past treatment, experts suggest lifelong surveillance for patients with a history of OPMDs.[94,110] The intervals between such surveillance visits vary depending on each patient's clinical course.

WHAT DOES THE FUTURE HOLD?

The molecular era has led to tremendous advances in understanding of the altered genetic and epigenetic landscape that drive carcinogenesis. It is the authors' hope and

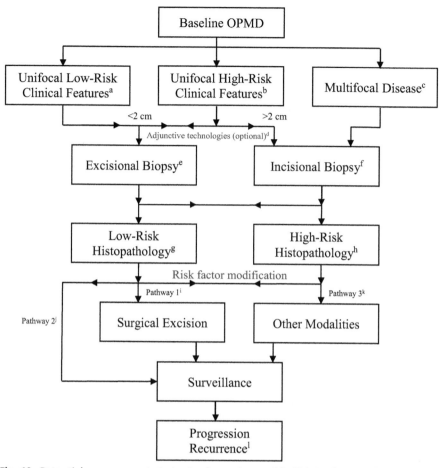

Fig. 10. Potential management strategies for patients with OPMDs. [a] Low-risk clinical features: homogeneous leukoplakia. [b] High-risk clinical features: nonhomogeneous leukoplakia, erythroplakia, erythroleukoplakia, and/or ulceration. [c] Multifocal disease: multisite lesions that are PVL. [d] Adjunctive techniques (optional, may be used if clinician has expertise): may facilitate biopsy site selection/margin determination. [e] Excisional biopsy: lesion <2 cm in diameter, accessible surgical site. [f] Incisional biopsy: lesion >2 cm, single site for homogeneous lesions(s); single or multiple sites for nonhomogeneous lesion(s). [g] Low-risk histopathology: epithelial hyperkeratosis/hyperplasia, verrucous hyperplasia, mild epithelial dysplasia. [h] High-risk histopathology: moderate-severe epithelial dysplasia, carcinoma-in-situ. Note: if OSCC, patient referred for oncologic management. [i] Pathway*1: initial surgical excision (unless lesion underwent baseline excision), that is, removal of visible lesion by cold blade, electrocautery, laser. This pathway is indicated preferably for lesions with high-risk pathology that are amenable to surgery, or optional for lesions with low-risk pathology. [j] Pathway* 2: initial surveillance, that is, monitoring those patients who (1) underwent successful baseline excisional biopsy with a diagnosis of either high or low-risk pathology, but with no residual lesion; (2) have a residual lesion or lesions after baseline biopsy with a diagnosis of low-risk pathology; or (3) have a residual lesion or lesions after baseline biopsy with a diagnosis of high-risk pathology that are not amenable to surgery. [k] Pathway* 3: other modalities, that is, PDT, chemoprevention, or other modalities as per experience of provider. [l] Progression/recurrence: clinical progression of existing OPMD, or recurrence of OPMD after treatment, warranting further diagnostic evaluation. If MT, patient referred for oncologic management. * Note: there are no evidence-based management pathways. In general, expert clinicians should manage all patients with a histopathologic finding of dysplasia (low risk and high risk), carcinoma in situ and OSCC.

expectation that these molecular advances will allow clinicians to improve risk stratification of patients with OPMDs, linking them to interventions commensurate with their risk profiles, particularly through the development of a genome atlas for OPMDs.[54,111] There would be justification for aggressive surgical/ablative treatment or systemic agents associated with toxicity (eg, chemotherapy, targeted therapy, or even immunotherapy) for patients with OPMDs at high risk for progression and MT. For those with a moderate-risk profile, a less aggressive approach is indicated, possibly including low-toxicity chemopreventive agents. The lowest-risk patients might be amenable to surveillance alone with periodic assessment for markers (histopathologic, cytopathologic, or other novel biomarker assessment). Translational research leading to the identification of agents that target important pathways of carcinogenesis are under development and in clinical trials. One drug currently under investigation is metformin, an oral hypoglycemic agent with an excellent safety profile, which has been shown in case-control studies to reduce the risk and prognosis of head and neck cancers,[112] and in animal studies to reduce the activity of the mammalian target of rapamycin complex 1 and lower the risk of MT.[113] Another promising drug, the anticonvulsant agent valproic acid, has been demonstrated to be a potent inhibitor of proliferation in vivo.[114]

Surgical excision performed in conjunction with adjuncts that can facilitate margin delineation (eg, optical detection methods, vital staining, or nanotechnologies with ligands that bind specifically to neoplastic cells) are also under investigation. Finally, surveillance of patients with a history OPMDs using emerging technologies (eg, live biopsies using high-resolution microendoscopy, optical coherence spectroscopy and other optical platforms, and point-of-care salivary or cytopathologic platforms using combinations of predictive biomarkers) could conceivably replace the need for invasive biopsy and histopathology and allow for improved monitoring. Yet, all these advances come with a price tag, and with current health care costs, it is hard to imagine these novel technologies will quickly move across all tiers of clinical care.

Study design is critical to the evaluation of new interventions. Adequately powered multicenter prospective RCTs with meaningful endpoints (ie, MTRs or validated surrogate markers) and sufficient follow-up are needed. Changes in habit use patterns during studies can confound study results and must be assessed.

SUMMARY

The management of patients with OPMDs must begin with modification of avoidable risk factors, such as tobacco use, heavy alcohol, and poor diet. Regression of OPMDs is possible with this strategy alone; however, follow-up is critical. Risk stratification based on the current paradigm of clinical and histopathologic factors dictates that patients with unifocal OPMDs with high-risk clinical features (ie, nonhomogeneous OLs [eg, erythroleukoplakias], OE, or persistent ulcers with no clear explanation) undergo incisional biopsy or biopsies to establish a baseline diagnosis. Such lesions often have variable histopathology and those diagnosed with moderate to severe dysplasia (or carcinoma in situ), if amenable in terms of size or accessibility, are strong candidates for surgical excision (with submission of the specimen for histopathologic evaluation, including margin assessment). Patients with unifocal OPMDs with low-risk features, such as well-circumscribed, small (ie, <200 mm^2), flat, homogeneous leukoplakias, typically have a diagnosis of mild or moderate epithelial dysplasia and are amenable to excisional biopsy at baseline. All patients with a history of dysplasia, similar to those with a history of OSCC, require close surveillance for recurrence or MT.

The challenge in patients with OPMDs is the management of those who recur despite baseline excision or those with multifocal disease, such as PVL with high rates of MT. Serial excisions are often fruitless, and expert clinicians typically resort to close surveillance to intercept early MT, followed by oncologic treatment. **Fig. 10** delineates potential management strategies for patients with OPMDs.

The role for other surgical/ablative modalities or chemopreventive agents is dictated by the experience and preference of the treating clinician, with appropriate informed consent to allow patients to understand the risks and benefits.

REFERENCES

1. Warnakulasuriya S, Johnson NW, van der Waal I. Nomenclature and classification of potentially malignant disorders of the oral mucosa. J Oral Pathol Med 2007;36(10):575–80.
2. van der Waal I. Potentially malignant disorders of the oral and oropharyngeal mucosa; terminology, classification and present concepts of management. Oral Oncol 2009;45(4–5):317–23.
3. van der Waal I. Oral potentially malignant disorders: is malignant transformation predictable and preventable? Med Oral Patol Oral Cir Bucal 2014;19(4): e386–90.
4. Villa A, Woo SB. Leukoplakia-A diagnostic and management algorithm. J Oral Maxillofac Surg 2017;75(4):723–34.
5. Kramer IR, Lucas RB, Pindborg JJ, et al. Definition of leukoplakia and related lesions: an aid to studies on oral precancer. Oral Surg Oral Med Oral Pathol 1978;46(4):518–39.
6. Warnakulasuriya S. Semi-quantitative clinical description of oral submucous fibrosis. Ann Dent 1987;46(2):18–21.
7. Roopashree MR, Gondhalekar RV, Shashikanth MC, et al. Pathogenesis of oral lichen planus–a review. J Oral Pathol Med 2010;39(10):729–34.
8. Amagasa T. Oral premalignant lesions. Int J Clin Oncol 2011;16(1):1–4.
9. Rajaraman P, Anderson BO, Basu P, et al. Recommendations for screening and early detection of common cancers in india. Lancet Oncol 2015;16(7):e352–61.
10. Tadakamadla J, Kumar S, Lalloo R, et al. Qualitative analysis of the impact of oral potentially malignant disorders on daily life activities. PLoS One 2017; 12(4):e0175531.
11. Bouquot JE. Oral leukoplakia and erythroplakia: a review and update. Pract Periodontics Aesthet Dent 1994;6(6):9–17 [quiz: 19].
12. Smith LW, Bhargava K, Mani NJ, et al. Oral cancer and precancerous lesions in 57,518 industrial workers of gujarat, india. Indian J Cancer 1975;12(2):118–23.
13. Petti S. Pooled estimate of world leukoplakia prevalence: a systematic review. Oral Oncol 2003;39(8):770–80.
14. Napier SS, Speight PM. Natural history of potentially malignant oral lesions and conditions: an overview of the literature. J Oral Pathol Med 2008;37(1):1–10.
15. Johnson NW, Jayasekara P, Amarasinghe AA. Squamous cell carcinoma and precursor lesions of the oral cavity: epidemiology and aetiology. Periodontol 2000 2011;57(1):19–37.
16. Warnakulasuriya S, Ariyawardana A. Malignant transformation of oral leukoplakia: a systematic review of observational studies. J Oral Pathol Med 2016; 45(3):155–66.

17. Mortazavi H, Baharvand M, Mehdipour M. Oral potentially malignant disorders: an overview of more than 20 entities. J Dent Res Dent Clin Dent Prospects 2014; 8(1):6–14.
18. Bhargava K, Smith LW, Mani NJ, et al. A follow up study of oral cancer and precancerous lesions in 57,518 industrial workers of gujarat, india. Indian J Cancer 1975;12(2):124–9.
19. Mehta FS, Shroff BC, Gupta PC, et al. Oral leukoplakia in relation to tobacco habits. A ten-year follow-up study of bombay policemen. Oral Surg Oral Med Oral Pathol 1972;34(3):426–33.
20. Arduino PG, Bagan J, El-Naggar AK, et al. Urban legends series: oral leukoplakia. Oral Dis 2013;19(7):642–59.
21. Scully C. Oral cancer aetiopathogenesis; past, present and future aspects. Med Oral Patol Oral Cir Bucal 2011;16(3):e306–11.
22. Amagasa T, Yamashiro M, Uzawa N. Oral premalignant lesions: from a clinical perspective. Int J Clin Oncol 2011;16(1):5–14.
23. Thomson PJ, McCaul JA, Ridout F, et al. To treat...or not to treat? clinicians' views on the management of oral potentially malignant disorders. Br J Oral Maxillofac Surg 2015;53(10):1027–31.
24. Pindborg JJ, Roed-Peterson B, Renstrup G. Role of smoking in floor of the mouth leukoplakias. J Oral Pathol 1972;1(1):22–9.
25. Reibel J. Prognosis of oral pre-malignant lesions: significance of clinical, histopathological, and molecular biological characteristics. Crit Rev Oral Biol Med 2003;14(1):47–62.
26. Gopinath D, Thannikunnath BV, Neermunda SF. Prevalence of carcinomatous foci in oral leukoplakia: a clinicopathologic study of 546 indian samples. J Clin Diagn Res 2016;10(8):ZC78–83.
27. Reichart PA, Philipsen HP. Oral erythroplakia–a review. Oral Oncol 2005;41(6): 551–61.
28. Shafer WG, Waldron CA. Erythroplakia of the oral cavity. Cancer 1975;36(3): 1021–8.
29. Hashibe M, Mathew B, Kuruvilla B, et al. Chewing tobacco, alcohol, and the risk of erythroplakia. Cancer Epidemiol Biomarkers Prev 2000;9(7):639–45.
30. Neville BW, Day TA. Oral cancer and precancerous lesions. CA Cancer J Clin 2002;52(4):195–215.
31. Bouquot JE, Ephros H. Erythroplakia: the dangerous red mucosa. Pract Periodontics Aesthet Dent 1995;7(6):59–67 [quiz: 68].
32. McCartan BE, Healy CM. The reported prevalence of oral lichen planus: a review and critique. J Oral Pathol Med 2008;37(8):447–53.
33. Ismail SB, Kumar SK, Zain RB. Oral lichen planus and lichenoid reactions: etiopathogenesis, diagnosis, management and malignant transformation. J Oral Sci 2007;49(2):89–106.
34. Fitzpatrick SG, Hirsch SA, Gordon SC. The malignant transformation of oral lichen planus and oral lichenoid lesions: a systematic review. J Am Dent Assoc 2014;145(1):45–56.
35. Aghbari SMH, Abushouk AI, Attia A, et al. Malignant transformation of oral lichen planus and oral lichenoid lesions: a meta-analysis of 20095 patient data. Oral Oncol 2017;68:92–102.
36. Arakeri G, Patil SG, Aljabab AS, et al. Oral submucous fibrosis: an update on pathophysiology of malignant transformation. J Oral Pathol Med 2017;46(6): 413–7.

37. Tilakaratne WM, Ekanayaka RP, Warnakulasuriya S. Oral submucous fibrosis: a historical perspective and a review on etiology and pathogenesis. Oral Surg Oral Med Oral Pathol Oral Radiol 2016;122(2):178–91.

38. Chaturvedi P, Malik A, Nair D, et al. Oral squamous cell carcinoma associated with oral submucous fibrosis have better oncologic outcome than those without. Oral Surg Oral Med Oral Pathol Oral Radiol 2017;124(3):225–30.

39. Mohiuddin S, Fatima N, Hosein S, et al. High risk of malignant transformation of oral submucous fibrosis in pakistani females: a potential national disaster. J Pak Med Assoc 2016;66(11):1362–6.

40. Murti PR, Bhonsle RB, Pindborg JJ, et al. Malignant transformation rate in oral submucous fibrosis over a 17-year period. Community Dent Oral Epidemiol 1985;13(6):340–1.

41. Hansen LS, Olson JA, Silverman S. Jr. Proliferative verrucous leukoplakia. A long-term study of thirty patients. Oral Surg Oral Med Oral Pathol 1985;60(3): 285–98.

42. Borgna SC, Clarke PT, Schache AG, et al. Management of proliferative verrucous leukoplakia: Justification for a conservative approach. Head Neck 2017; 39(10):1997–2003.

43. Capella DL, Goncalves JM, Abrantes AAA, et al. Proliferative verrucous leukoplakia: diagnosis, management and current advances. Braz J Otorhinolaryngol 2017;83(5):585–93.

44. Batsakis JG, Suarez P, el-Naggar AK. Proliferative verrucous leukoplakia and its related lesions. Oral Oncol 1999;35(4):354–9.

45. Gillenwater AM, Vigneswaran N, Fatani H, et al. Proliferative verrucous leukoplakia: recognition and differentiation from conventional leukoplakia and mimics. Head Neck 2014;36(11):1662–8.

46. Bagan JV, Jimenez Y, Sanchis JM, et al. Proliferative verrucous leukoplakia: high incidence of gingival squamous cell carcinoma. J Oral Pathol Med 2003;32(7): 379–82.

47. Silverman S Jr, Gorsky M, Lozada F. Oral leukoplakia and malignant transformation. A follow-up study of 257 patients. Cancer 1984;53(3):563–8.

48. Bagan JV, Jimenez-Soriano Y, Diaz-Fernandez JM, et al. Malignant transformation of proliferative verrucous leukoplakia to oral squamous cell carcinoma: a series of 55 cases. Oral Oncol 2011;47(8):732–5.

49. Campisi G, Giovannelli L, Ammatuna P, et al. Proliferative verrucous vs conventional leukoplakia: no significantly increased risk of HPV infection. Oral Oncol 2004;40(8):835–40.

50. Scully C. Challenges in predicting which oral mucosal potentially malignant disease will progress to neoplasia. Oral Dis 2014;20(1):1–5.

51. Holmstrup P, Vedtofte P, Reibel J, et al. Long-term treatment outcome of oral premalignant lesions. Oral Oncol 2006;42(5):461–74.

52. Mehanna HM, Rattay T, Smith J, et al. Treatment and follow-up of oral dysplasia - a systematic review and meta-analysis. Head Neck 2009;31(12):1600–9.

53. Alaizari NA, Sperandio M, Odell EW, et al. Meta-analysis of the predictive value of DNA aneuploidy in malignant transformation of oral potentially malignant disorders. J Oral Pathol Med 2017. [Epub ahead of print].

54. Monteiro de Oliveira Novaes JA, William WN Jr. Prognostic factors, predictive markers and cancer biology: the triad for successful oral cancer chemoprevention. Future Oncol 2016;12(20):2379–86.

55. Speight PM, Epstein J, Kujan O, et al. Screening for oral cancer-a perspective from the global oral cancer forum. Oral Surg Oral Med Oral Pathol Oral Radiol 2017;123(6):680–7.

56. Moyer VA, U.S. Preventive Services Task Force. Screening for oral cancer: U.S. preventive services task force recommendation statement. Ann Intern Med 2014;160(1):55–60.

57. AAOM clinical practice statement: subject: oral cancer examination and screening. Oral Surg Oral Med Oral Pathol Oral Radiol 2016;122(2):174–5.

58. Rethman MP, Carpenter W, Cohen EE, et al. Evidence-based clinical recommendations regarding screening for oral squamous cell carcinomas. J Am Dent Assoc 2010;141(5):509–20.

59. Epstein JB. Screening for oral potentially malignant epithelial lesions and squamous cell carcinoma: a discussion of benefit and risk. J Can Dent Assoc 2014; 80:e47.

60. Epstein JB, Gorsky M, Cabay RJ, et al. Screening for and diagnosis of oral premalignant lesions and oropharyngeal squamous cell carcinoma: role of primary care physicians. Can Fam Physician 2008;54(6):870–5.

61. Tadakamadla J, Kumar S, Johnson NW. Quality of life in patients with oral potentially malignant disorders: a systematic review. Oral Surg Oral Med Oral Pathol Oral Radiol 2015;119(6):644–55.

62. Tadakamadla J, Kumar S, Lalloo R, et al. Development and validation of a quality-of-life questionnaire for patients with oral potentially malignant disorders. Oral Surg Oral Med Oral Pathol Oral Radiol 2017;123(3):338–49.

63. Barnes L, Eveson J, Reichart P, et al. World health organizations classification of tumour. In: IARC Press, editor. Pathology & genetics of head and neck tumours. Lyon (France): IARC Press; 2005. p. 177–8.

64. Abbey LM, Kaugars GE, Gunsolley JC, et al. Intraexaminer and interexaminer reliability in the diagnosis of oral epithelial dysplasia. Oral Surg Oral Med Oral Pathol Oral Radiol Endod 1995;80(2):188–91.

65. Geetha KM, Leeky M, Narayan TV, et al. Grading of oral epithelial dysplasia: points to ponder. J Oral Maxillofac Pathol 2015;19(2):198–204.

66. Dionne KR, Warnakulasuriya S, Zain RB, et al. Potentially malignant disorders of the oral cavity: current practice and future directions in the clinic and laboratory. Int J Cancer 2015;136(3):503–15.

67. Macey R, Walsh T, Brocklehurst P, et al. Diagnostic tests for oral cancer and potentially malignant disorders in patients presenting with clinically evident lesions. Cochrane Database Syst Rev 2015;(5):CD010276.

68. Patton LL, Epstein JB, Kerr AR. Adjunctive techniques for oral cancer examination and lesion diagnosis: a systematic review of the literature. J Am Dent Assoc 2008;139(7):896–905 [quiz: 993–4].

69. Lingen MW, Kalmar JR, Karrison T, et al. Critical evaluation of diagnostic aids for the detection of oral cancer. Oral Oncol 2008;44(1):10–22.

70. Rethman MP, Carpenter W, Cohen EE, et al. Evidence-based clinical recommendations regarding screening for oral squamous cell carcinomas. Tex Dent J 2012;129(5):491–507.

71. Warnakulasuriya S, Kerr AR. Oral submucous fibrosis: a review of the current management and possible directions for novel therapies. Oral Surg Oral Med Oral Pathol Oral Radiol 2016;122(2):232–41.

72. Lodi G, Carrozzo M, Furness S, et al. Interventions for treating oral lichen planus: a systematic review. Br J Dermatol 2012;166(5):938–47.

73. Roosaar A, Yin L, Johansson AL, et al. A long-term follow-up study on the natural course of oral leukoplakia in a swedish population-based sample. J Oral Pathol Med 2007;36(2):78–82.

74. Gupta PC, Murti PR, Bhonsle RB, et al. Effect of cessation of tobacco use on the incidence of oral mucosal lesions in a 10-yr follow-up study of 12,212 users. Oral Dis 1995;1(1):54–8.

75. Martin GC, Brown JP, Eifler CW, et al. Oral leukoplakia status six weeks after cessation of smokeless tobacco use. J Am Dent Assoc 1999;130(7):945–54.

76. Roed-Petersen B. Effect on oral leukoplakia of reducing or ceasing tobacco smoking. Acta Derm Venereol 1982;62(2):164–7.

77. Vladimirov BS, Schiodt M. The effect of quitting smoking on the risk of unfavorable events after surgical treatment of oral potentially malignant lesions. Int J Oral Maxillofac Surg 2009;38(11):1188–93.

78. Clinical Practice Guideline Treating Tobacco Use and Dependence 2008 Update Panel, Liaisons, and Staff. A clinical practice guideline for treating tobacco use and dependence: 2008 update. A U.S. public health service report. Am J Prev Med 2008;35(2):158–76.

79. Willenbring ML, Massey SH, Gardner MB. Helping patients who drink too much: an evidence-based guide for primary care clinicians. Am Fam Physician 2009; 80(1):44–50.

80. Lodi G, Franchini R, Warnakulasuriya S, et al. Interventions for treating oral leukoplakia to prevent oral cancer. Cochrane Database Syst Rev 2016;(7):CD001829.

81. Sankaranarayanan R, Mathew B, Varghese C, et al. Chemoprevention of oral leukoplakia with vitamin A and beta carotene: an assessment. Oral Oncol 1997;33(4):231–6.

82. Nagao T, Warnakulasuriya S, Nakamura T, et al. Treatment of oral leukoplakia with a low-dose of beta-carotene and vitamin C supplements: a randomized controlled trial. Int J Cancer 2015;136(7):1708–17.

83. Stich HF, Hornby AP, Mathew B, et al. Response of oral leukoplakias to the administration of vitamin A. Cancer Lett 1988;40(1):93–101.

84. Singh M, Krishanappa R, Bagewadi A, et al. Efficacy of oral lycopene in the treatment of oral leukoplakia. Oral Oncol 2004;40(6):591–6.

85. Epstein JB, Wong FL, Millner A, et al. Topical bleomycin treatment of oral leukoplakia: a randomized double-blind clinical trial. Head Neck 1994;16(6):539–44.

86. Hong WK, Endicott J, Itri LM, et al. 13-cis-retinoic acid in the treatment of oral leukoplakia. N Engl J Med 1986;315(24):1501–5.

87. Li N, Sun Z, Han C, et al. The chemopreventive effects of tea on human oral precancerous mucosa lesions. Proc Soc Exp Biol Med 1999;220(4):218–24.

88. Mallery SR, Tong M, Shumway BS, et al. Topical application of a mucoadhesive freeze-dried black raspberry gel induces clinical and histologic regression and reduces loss of heterozygosity events in premalignant oral intraepithelial lesions: results from a multicentered, placebo-controlled clinical trial. Clin Cancer Res 2014;20(7):1910–24.

89. William WN Jr, Papadimitrakopoulou V, Lee JJ, et al. Erlotinib and the risk of oral cancer: the erlotinib prevention of oral cancer (EPOC) randomized clinical trial. JAMA Oncol 2016;2(2):209–16.

90. Goralczyk R. Beta-carotene and lung cancer in smokers: review of hypotheses and status of research. Nutr Cancer 2009;61(6):767–74.

91. Slaughter DP, Southwick HW, Smejkal W. Field cancerization in oral stratified squamous epithelium; clinical implications of multicentric origin. Cancer 1953; 6(5):963–8.

92. Braakhuis BJ, Tabor MP, Kummer JA, et al. A genetic explanation of slaughter's concept of field cancerization: evidence and clinical implications. Cancer Res 2003;63(8):1727–30.
93. Abadie WM, Partington EJ, Fowler CB, et al. Optimal management of proliferative verrucous leukoplakia: a systematic review of the literature. Otolaryngol Head Neck Surg 2015;153(4):504–11.
94. Holmstrup P, Dabelsteen E. Oral leukoplakia-to treat or not to treat. Oral Dis 2016;22(6):494–7.
95. Arduino PG, Surace A, Carbone M, et al. Outcome of oral dysplasia: a retrospective hospital-based study of 207 patients with a long follow-up. J Oral Pathol Med 2009;38(6):540–4.
96. Tambuwala A, Sangle A, Khan A, et al. Excision of oral leukoplakia by CO2 lasers versus traditional scalpel: a comparative study. J Maxillofac Oral Surg 2014;13(3):320–7.
97. Lopez-Jornet P, Camacho-Alonso F. Comparison of pain and swelling after removal of oral leukoplakia with CO(2) laser and cold knife: a randomized clinical trial. Med Oral Patol Oral Cir Bucal 2013;18(1):e38–44.
98. Broccoletti R, Cafaro A, Gambino A, et al. Er:YAG laser versus cold knife excision in the treatment of nondysplastic oral lesions: a randomized comparative study for the postoperative period. Photomed Laser Surg 2015;33(12):604–9.
99. Mogedas-Vegara A, Hueto-Madrid JA, Chimenos-Kustner E, et al. Oral leukoplakia treatment with the carbon dioxide laser: a systematic review of the literature. J Craniomaxillofac Surg 2016;44(4):331–6.
100. Thomson PJ, Goodson ML, Cocks K, et al. Interventional laser surgery for oral potentially malignant disorders: a longitudinal patient cohort study. Int J Oral Maxillofac Surg 2017;46(3):337–42.
101. Yang SW, Tsai CN, Lee YS, et al. Treatment outcome of dysplastic oral leukoplakia with carbon dioxide laser–emphasis on the factors affecting recurrence. J Oral Maxillofac Surg 2011;69(6):e78–87.
102. Chandu A, Smith AC. The use of CO2 laser in the treatment of oral white patches: outcomes and factors affecting recurrence. Int J Oral Maxillofac Surg 2005;34(4):396–400.
103. Chainani-Wu N, Madden E, Cox D, et al. Toluidine blue aids in detection of dysplasia and carcinoma in suspicious oral lesions. Oral Dis 2015;21(7):879–85.
104. Yu CH, Lin HP, Cheng SJ, et al. Cryotherapy for oral precancers and cancers. J Formos Med Assoc 2014;113(5):272–7.
105. Kawczyk-Krupka A, Waskowska J, Raczkowska-Siostrzonek A, et al. Comparison of cryotherapy and photodynamic therapy in treatment of oral leukoplakia. Photodiagnosis Photodyn Ther 2012;9(2):148–55.
106. Saini R, Poh CF. Photodynamic therapy: a review and its prospective role in the management of oral potentially malignant disorders. Oral Dis 2013;19(5):440–51.
107. Vohra F, Al-Kheraif AA, Qadri T, et al. Efficacy of photodynamic therapy in the management of oral premalignant lesions. A systematic review. Photodiagnosis Photodyn Ther 2015;12(1):150–9.
108. Gondivkar SM, Gadbail AR, Choudhary MG, et al. Photodynamic treatment outcomes of potentially-malignant lesions and malignancies of the head and neck region: a systematic review. J Investig Clin Dent 2017. [Epub ahead of print].
109. Jerjes W, Upile T, Hamdoon Z, et al. Photodynamic therapy outcome for oral dysplasia. Lasers Surg Med 2011;43(3):192–9.

110. Ho MW, Field EA, Field JK, et al. Outcomes of oral squamous cell carcinoma arising from oral epithelial dysplasia: rationale for monitoring premalignant oral lesions in a multidisciplinary clinic. Br J Oral Maxillofac Surg 2013;51(7): 594–9.

111. Bauman JE, Grandis J. Oral cancer chemoprevention–the end of EPOC, the beginning of an epoch of molecular selection. JAMA Oncol 2016;2(2):178–9.

112. Rego DF, Pavan LM, Elias ST, et al. Effects of metformin on head and neck cancer: a systematic review. Oral Oncol 2015;51(5):416–22.

113. Vitale-Cross L, Molinolo AA, Martin D, et al. Metformin prevents the development of oral squamous cell carcinomas from carcinogen-induced premalignant lesions. Cancer Prev Res (Phila) 2012;5(4):562–73.

114. Gan CP, Hamid S, Hor SY, et al. Valproic acid: growth inhibition of head and neck cancer by induction of terminal differentiation and senescence. Head Neck 2012;34(3):344–53.

115. Piattelli A, Fioroni M, Santinelli A, et al. Bcl-2 expression and apoptotic bodies in 13-cis-retinoic acid (isotretinoin)-topically treated oral leukoplakia: a pilot study. Oral Oncol 1999;35(3):314–20.

116. Tsao AS, Liu D, Martin J, et al. Phase II randomized, placebo-controlled trial of green tea extract in patients with high-risk oral premalignant lesions. Cancer Prev Res (Phila) 2009;2(11):931–41.

117. Sun Z, Guan X, Li N, et al. Chemoprevention of oral cancer in animal models, and effect on leukoplakias in human patients with ZengShengPing, a mixture of medicinal herbs. Oral Oncol 2010;46(2):105–10.

118. Armstrong WB, Taylor TH, Kennedy AR, et al. Bowman birk inhibitor concentrate and oral leukoplakia: a randomized phase IIb trial. Cancer Prev Res (Phila) 2013;6(5):410–8.

119. Mulshine JL, Atkinson JC, Greer RO, et al. Randomized, double-blind, placebo-controlled phase IIb trial of the cyclooxygenase inhibitor ketorolac as an oral rinse in oropharyngeal leukoplakia. Clin Cancer Res 2004;10(5):1565–73.

120. Papadimitrakopoulou VA, William WN Jr, Dannenberg AJ, et al. Pilot randomized phase II study of celecoxib in oral premalignant lesions. Clin Cancer Res 2008; 14(7):2095–101.

Oral Cancer
Genetics and the Role of Precision Medicine

Chia-Cheng Li, DDS, DMSc[a],*, Zhen Shen, PhD[b],
Roxanne Bavarian, DMD[b,c], Fan Yang, DDS, PhD[b],
Aditi Bhattacharya, BDS, MDS, PhD[d]

KEYWORDS

- Oral cancer • Oral squamous cell carcinoma • Malignant transformation
- Epigenetics • Omics technology • Big data • Personalized medicine
- Precision medicine

KEY POINTS

- Oral squamous cell carcinoma (OSCC), a distinct subtype of head and neck squamous cell carcinoma, is typically human papillomavirus-negative and harbors *TP53* loss-of-function mutations.
- OSCC is thought to begin with cancer initiating cells that are able to self-renew and generate heterogeneous clones of neoplastic cells to comprise the tumor (ie, tumor heterogeneity).
- Carcinogenesis is a multistep process, which involves an accumulation of both genetic and epigenetic alterations in oncogenes and/or tumor suppressor genes.
- Metastasis is one of the major prognostic indicators in OSCC. Both epithelial-to-mesenchymal transition and interactions between OSCC cells and the tumor microenvironment play significant roles in this complex process.
- The integration of omics technologies, bioinformatics, and molecular biology uncovers complex, clinically meaningful information that greatly improves our understanding of the disease process.

INTRODUCTION TO ORAL CANCER

Cancer is a major global health issue. According to the GLOBOCAN project of the International Agency for Research on Cancer, there were approximately 14.1 million newly

[a] Department of Oral Medicine, Infection and Immunity, Harvard School of Dental Medicine, 188 Longwood Avenue, Boston, MA 02115, USA; [b] Harvard School of Dental Medicine, 188 Longwood Avenue, Boston, MA 02115, USA; [c] Division of Oral Medicine and Dentistry, Brigham and Women's Hospital, Francis Street, Boston, MA 02115, USA; [d] Department of Oral and Maxillofacial Surgery, NYU College of Dentistry, East 24th Street, New York, NY 10010, USA
* Corresponding author.
E-mail address: Chia-Cheng_Li@hsdm.harvard.edu

Dent Clin N Am 62 (2018) 29–46
http://dx.doi.org/10.1016/j.cden.2017.08.002
0011-8532/18/© 2017 Elsevier Inc. All rights reserved.

diagnosed cancer cases with 8.2 million deaths worldwide in 2012.[1] Globally, oral cancer is one of the leading cancers, accounting for 2% of all cancer cases, with a nearly 50% mortality rate.[1] Internationally, the highest rates of oral cancer are seen in South Asian countries, such as Sri Lanka, India, and Taiwan, which are attributed to the high rates of cigarette smoking and areca nut use in these countries.[2] In the United States, 48,330 cases of oral and oropharyngeal cancer are diagnosed each year, comprising approximately 3% of all cancer cases.[3–8] It is the eighth leading cancer in men, with more than two-thirds of oral cancer cases occurring in male patients.[1,3]

Multiple factors contribute to the initiation of oral cancer. In addition to the well-established roles of tobacco, alcohol, and areca nut as risk factors for oral cancer, high-risk human papillomavirus infection (eg, HPV-16 and HPV-18) has been identified as a significant risk factor for oropharyngeal cancer.[9] Recent studies over the past decade have revealed an increasing incidence of HPV-positive oropharyngeal cancer in developed countries, which exhibits a better prognosis than HPV-negative oral cancer.[10,11] Specific germline mutations are also associated with a higher incidence of oral cancer. For example, patients with Li-Fraumeni syndrome (germline TP53 mutation) are predisposed to early-onset oral cancer.[12] Additionally, patients with Fanconi anemia, a condition characterized by defects in the DNA repair process and consequent chromosomal instability, are associated with aggressive oral cancers that present at a young age.[13,14] Due to defective telomerase maintenance, patients with dyskeratosis congenita exhibit a thousand-fold increased risk for developing oral cancer.[15]

Squamous cell carcinoma (SCC) constitutes more than 90% of all cancer cases arising in the head and neck region, including the oral cavity and oropharynx.[16] Oral cancer and oropharyngeal cancer are two distinctive entities clinically, histopathologically, and genetically.[17] This article focuses on oral cancer. The most common sites of oral SCC (OSCC) are the tongue and floor of mouth, which account for more than 50% of all the cases, followed by the gingiva, palatal mucosa, and buccal and labial mucosa.[18] OSCC usually progresses rapidly, and the prognosis is closely associated with the tumor staging.[19] In the United States, approximately 50% of the OSCC patients present with regional or distant metastasis at the time of diagnosis.[20] OSCC tumors can double in size within three months, which clinically equates to a T1 tumor progressing to a T3 tumor in less than two years.[21] This accelerated progression corresponds to a dismal prognosis. The overall 5-year survival rate of OSCC is approximately 60%, varying between 80% for stage I cancers and 40% for stage IV cancers.[3]

Treatment strategies for OSCC vary based on the stage at time of diagnosis. Patients with localized disease typically receive surgery and/or radiotherapy, leading to a high probability of long-term survival but with considerable morbidity.[22] With metastatic OSCC, chemotherapy and radiotherapy are the mainstays of treatment.[22] Recently, targeted therapeutics have been introduced into treatment regimens or ongoing clinical trials to improve survival rate and reduce toxicity, such as cetuximab (monoclonal epidermal growth factor receptor [EGFR] antibody), bevacizumab (monoclonal vascular endothelial growth factor [VEGF] antibody), and mechanistic target of rapamycin (mTOR) inhibitors.[22] With the advancement of immunotherapy, monoclonal antibodies that target programmed cell death protein-1 (PD-1), a receptor of the immune escape pathway, such as nivolumab and pembrolizumab, have been approved by the Food and Drug Administration (FDA) for recurrent and/or metastatic head and neck SCC.[22]

Despite the progress in investigating the pathobiological mechanisms of OSCC, the prognosis has unfortunately not improved over the past few decades.[23] This is largely due to the frequent occurrence of local and regional OSCC recurrences as well as high morbidity and mortality rates.[23] The clinical challenge remains in accurately detecting regional metastasis and efficiently treating second primary OSCC and recurrent tumors.[23] This article reviews our understanding of the etiopathologic mechanisms of OSCC from both genetic and epigenetic perspectives and discusses the role of precision medicine in OSCC prevention, detection, and management.

INITIATION AND PROGRESSION OF ORAL SQUAMOUS CELL CARCINOMA
Initiation of Oral Squamous Cell Carcinoma—Field Cancerization

Most OSCC tumors develop from an existing premalignant lesion, such as leukoplakia, erythroplakia, or proliferative verrucous leukoplakia.[24] In addition, OSCC is notorious for its high recurrence rate and the frequent occurrence of synchronous and/or metachronous primary tumors.[23] To explain this clinical phenomenon and aid our understanding of OSCC initiation, Slaughter and colleagues[25] proposed the concept of "field cancerization." Field cancerization refers to the formation of large, preneoplastic fields of carcinogen-exposed mucosal epithelium that are not apparent on clinical or histologic examination. The process of field cancerization occurs at the molecular level. Cells acquire and accumulate a series of genetic or epigenetic alterations that lead to cell cycle dysregulation and uncontrolled cell proliferation, ultimately predisposing these cells toward malignant transformation.[24]

Field cancerization is a multistep process and has been described in many organ systems, such as oral epithelium, esophagus, and skin.[26,27] The precancerized fields in OSCC have been characterized based on the expression of a mutated tumor suppressor, p53.[27] This is caused by loss-of-function mutations of the gene *TP53* that encodes the tumor protein p53.[27] Initially, cells with *TP53* loss-of-function mutation form a patch, suggesting its clonal nature. These patches gradually expand by acquiring additional mutations, allowing for advantages toward cell proliferation, and eventually form a confluent preneoplastic field that displaces the normal epithelium.[28]

Initiation of Oral Squamous Cell Carcinoma—Cancer-initiating Cells in Oral Squamous Cell Carcinoma

Similar to other solid tumors, OSCC exhibits tumor heterogeneity.[29] OSCC is thought to begin with a specialized population of cancer-initiating cells (CICs)/cancer stem cells (CSCs), which possess stemness, or the ability to self-renew and generate heterogeneous clones of neoplastic cells that form a precancerized field and ultimately comprise the tumor.[30,31] Multiple hypotheses have been proposed to explain the origin of CICs, such as epigenetically altered normal tissue stem cells or dedifferentiated tumor cells.[32] More research needs to be done to clarify the origin of CICs in OSCC. CICs are slow-cycling cells and are resistant to conventional chemotherapeutics that target highly proliferative cells.[33] Thus, CICs are able to avoid cell death after chemotherapy and utilize their stem cell–like features to regenerate the whole tumor mass and cause a recurrence.[24,30]

Putative CICs of OSCCs have been defined by cell surface markers (eg, CD133 and CD44) or based on Hoechst dye exclusion (eg, side population), followed by xenograft transplantation assays.[33–36] These experiments, however, only demonstrated the ability of a defined population of OSCC cells to form tumors in a new environment and did not necessarily recapitulate the behavior of such cancer cells in their native environment. Thus, these studies provided little molecular insight into the mechanism by which CICs self-renew or differentiate into different cancer clones. Studies suggest that CICs can be more accurately defined and studied in intact tumors by lineage tracing and clonal analysis.[37–39] This in vivo approach typically involves a Cre recombinase-based cell type-specific fluorescent labeling. Cancer cells can be permanently labeled and tracked based on known stem cell markers (eg, Lgr5 promoter for intestinal crypt stem cells).[40] B-cell specific Moloney murine leukemia virus insertion site 1 (Bmi1), a transcription repressor, plays a critical role in cell senescence.[41] By applying the lineage tracing strategy, Bmi1$^+$ cells can be visualized in the basal cell layer of normal lingual epithelium, regulating tissue maintenance and regeneration.[42] Recent studies revealed that Bmi1$^+$ subpopulation in OSCC was a subset of slow-cycling tumor propagating cells and mediated invasive growth and regional metastasis of OSCC.[43,44] Eliminating Bmi1$^+$ OSCC cells significantly reduced the occurrence of metastasis, indicating the potential therapeutic value of Bmi1 inhibitors in OSCC treatments.[44]

Multistep Progression of Oral Squamous Cell Carcinoma

The multistep progression of OSCC involves an accumulation of both genetic and epigenetic alterations in oncogenes or tumor suppressor genes, leading to cell cycle dysregulation, inhibition of growth suppressors, and resistance to apoptosis (**Fig. 1**).[45,46] Meanwhile, the interactions between tumor cells and microenvironment enhance the progression and invasion of OSCC.

The role of chromosomal instability (eg, telomerase dysfunction and loss of heterozygosity [LOH]) in the process of malignant transformation has been studied extensively.[46] Telomeres are G-rich proteins at the distal ends of chromosomes that play a critical role in maintaining cell cycle homeostasis.[47] Telomerase is a telomere-specific polymerase that maintains telomere integrity by its functional subunit, telomerase reverse transcriptase (TERT), to synthesize the telomere sequences.[47] Mutations of TERT, which have been detected in 80% of OSCC tumors, lead to cell cycle dysregulation and uncontrolled cell proliferation.[48] It is unclear, however, if there is an association between TERT mutations and patient outcome. In addition to telomerase dysfunction, LOH of chromosomes 3p, 8p, 9p (p16), and 17p (p53) are often key events in OSCC initiation and progression.[48] LOH refers to the loss of chromosomal regions containing a gene (eg, tumor suppressor gene) in either the maternal or paternal allele, resulting in higher tumor susceptibility.[48] Specifically, LOH at 17p13 (p53 locus) is significantly associated with the higher incidence of OSCC development.[49] *TP53* gene, known as the "guardian of the genome," plays an essential role in cell cycle regulation and DNA damage-induced apoptosis (**Fig. 2**).[48,50] Up to 80% of OSCC tumors exhibit *TP53* inactivation, typically through point mutations, which are single-nucleotide mutations in the DNA sequence.[51,52] Inactivation of p53 can further cause cell immortalization.[53] Mutations of *CDKN2A*, *CCND1*, *PIK3CA*, *PTEN*, and *HRAS* can also cause cell cycle dysregulation and immortalization, and are associated with OSCC initiation and progression (see **Fig. 2**).[50–52] The tumor suppressor gene, *CDKN2A*, encodes the p16 protein that regulates cell cycle progression.[54] Deletion or inactivation of *CDKN2A* is associated with cell immortalization and is seen in approximately 50% of OSCC tumors.[54] Cyclin D1, a protein encoded by the *CCND1* gene, allows for progression through the cell cycle.[53] *CCND1* amplification leads to cell proliferation and is identified in 20% to 30% of OSCCs.[52,54] Upon binding with its ligand, EGFR, a transmembrane receptor tyrosine kinase, functions to regulate cell proliferation, survival, and apoptosis via multiple downstream signaling pathways (eg, PI3K/AKT pathway and Ras/Raf/mitogen-activated protein kinase [MAPK] pathway).[55,56] PIK3CA, a catalytic subunit of phosphatidylinositol 3-kinases (PI3K), is recruited by EGFR to activate the downstream survival cascade. The activity of PI3K is regulated by the tumor suppressor, phosphatase and tensin homolog (PTEN).[56] Inactivated or deleted PTEN enhances cell survival, migration, and angiogenesis via PIK3CA and AKT activation.[48] Amplification of PIK3CA and EGFR is present in 27% and 14% of OSCC tumors, respectively.[54,57] In addition, *NOTCH1*

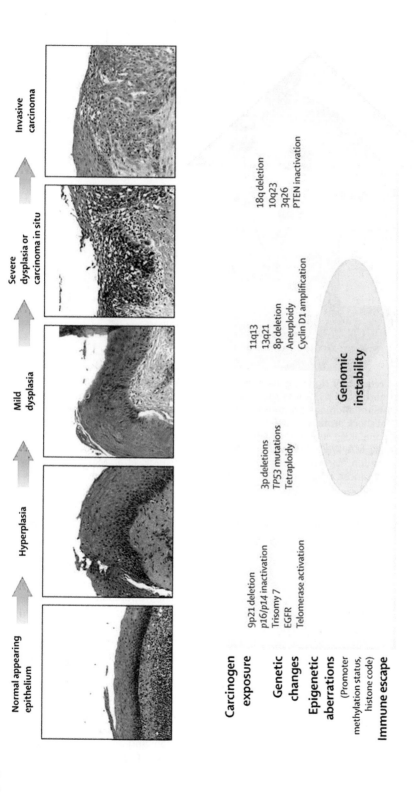

Fig. 1. Oral carcinogenesis is a complex multistep process characterized by an accumulation of genetic and epigenetic alterations, leading to genomic instability.[45] Histopathologic progression of OSCC is presented in hematoxylin-eosin stain (×200).[45] (*From* Agriris A, Karamouzis MV, Raben D, et al. Head and neck cancer. Lancet 2008;371[9625]:1696; with permission.)

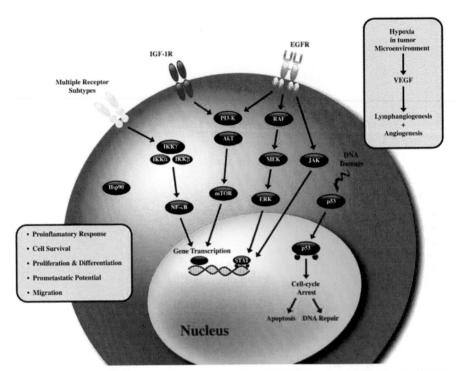

Fig. 2. Altered regulatory signaling pathways (eg, PI3K/AKT pathway and Ras/Raf/MAPK pathway) and inactivated p53 cause cell-cycle dysregulation and cell immortalization and contribute to the initiation and progression of OSCC.[50] ERK, extracellular signal–related kinase; Hsp90, heat shock protein 90; IGF-1R, insulinlike growth factor-1 receptor; IKKα, inhibitor κB kinase alpha; IKKβ, inhibitor κB kinase beta; IKKγ, inhibitor κB kinase gamma; JAK, Janus kinase; MEK, MAPK/ERK kinase; NF, nuclear factor; STAT, signal transducers and activators of transcription.[50] (*From* Stadler ME, Patel MR, Couch ME, et al. Molecular biology of head and neck cancer: risks and pathways. Hematol Oncol Clin North Am 2008;22:1106, vii; with permission.)

loss-of-function mutations are detected in 15% of OSCC tumors.[51,52,54] NOTCH1 regulates skin differentiation and homeostasis, and conditional *NOTCH1* knockout mice develop skin tumors, indicating its role as a tumor suppressor protein.[58]

Epigenetic alterations, such as DNA methylation and histone modifications, regulate gene expression by adjusting chromosomal structures as opposed to changing the DNA sequence.[59] Aberrant promoter hypermethylation interrupts the binding of transcription factors to the promoter of key tumor suppressor genes, leading to silencing of these genes and promotion of tumor growth.[60,61] Transcriptional silencing of the tumor suppressor gene, p16, is detected in 50% to 75% of OSCC tumors.[62–64] Many epigenetic drugs have been developed to effectively reverse DNA methylation that occurs in cancer. DNA methylation inhibitors were the first epigenetic drugs proposed for use as cancer therapeutics.[65] Research has also shown global DNA hypomethylation in OSCC tumors despite the regional promoter hypermethylation.[66] Moreover, the degree of global hypomethylation is enhanced in the advanced stage of OSCC.[66] Histones are structural proteins that are packaged with DNA into a complex organization. Histone modifications, such as acetylation and methylation, induce conformational changes of DNA molecules and regulate the transcriptional activities by either exposing or blocking the binding sites of transcription factors.[67] Aberrant histone modifications may lead to the abnormal transcriptional activity and contribute to malignant transformation (**Fig. 3**).[67,68] For example, recent studies revealed that hypoacetylation of H3K9ac is associated with cell proliferation and epithelial-to-mesenchymal transition (EMT) in OSCC.[69]

In addition to genetic and epigenetic alterations, microRNAs (miRNAs) contribute to oncogenesis by altering the expression of tumor suppressor genes and/or oncogenes.[70] The significance of miRNAs as a group of robust prognostic indicators in human cancers has long been recognized.[71] Molecular characterization of OSCCs based on 61 miRNAs achieved 93% accuracy to distinguish normal and malignant mucosal epithelium.[72] miRNAs are 18–23 nucleotide-long, single-stranded, noncoding RNAs that function as post-transcriptional repressors of their target genes.[73] The mechanisms that alter miRNA expression include transcriptional dysregulation, epigenetic modifications, chromosomal changes, single nucleotide polymorphisms (SNPs), and defects in the processing machinery.[74,75] An miRNA may regulate the expression of multiple targeted mRNA molecules.[76] Many altered miRNAs have been linked with the pathogenesis of OSCC.[70] For example, down-regulation of miR-375 is commonly seen in OSCC, and functional restoration of miR-375 can significantly suppress tumor aggressiveness, suggesting its role as a tumor suppressor.[70]

METASTASIS OF ORAL SQUAMOUS CELL CARCINOMA

Metastasis of cancer cells is one of the major prognostic indicators in OSCC.[46] Typically, metastatic tumors of OSCC present in the cervical lymph nodes and are

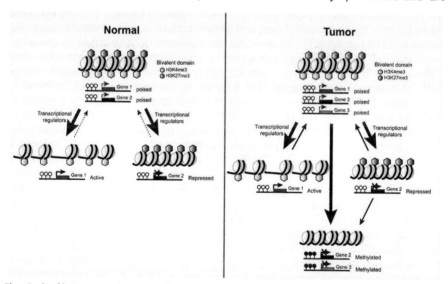

Fig. 3. (*Left*) In normal stem cells, many genes remain bivalent marks (ie, both active [H3K4me3] and repressed [H3K27me3]) at the promoter regions on the chromosomes. During normal development, this poised state will transform into either an active or repressed state to regulate gene expression. (*Right*) In cancer cells, the determined state can be reversed to bivalent state, and cells regain cellular plasticity (ie, dedifferentiation). In certain differentiation-related genes, the promoters are hypermethylated, leading to a permanently silenced state.[68] (*From* Easwaran H, Tsai HC, Baylin SB. Cancer epigenetics: tumor heterogeneity, plasticity of stem-like states, and drug resistance. Mol Cell 2014;54:720; with permission.)

associated with poor clinical prognosis.[46,77] The model of EMT provides an appealing hypothesis to explain this extremely complex multistep process.[78] EMT refers to the transdifferentiation program of epithelial cells into motile mesenchymal cells that allow for growth and invasion. With the loss of cell polarity and cell-cell adhesion molecules (eg, E-cadherin), OSCC cells acquire mesenchymal features, such as motile phenotypes and expression of mesenchymal markers (eg, N-cadherin and vimentin).[78] In addition, there are constant interactions between OSCC cells and the surrounding microenvironment that also promote metastasis.[79]

Although the molecular mechanism of EMT is not yet fully understood, it is known to rely on paracrine signaling between the tumor cells and the surrounding tumor microenvironment (TME).[80] The TME is composed of stromal cells, immune cells, and the surrounding extracellular matrix (ECM).[80] One of the most prominent and extensively studied signaling pathways associated with EMT is the transforming growth factor β (TGF-β) pathway. TGF-β functions by binding to TGF-β receptors I and II, which are serine/threonine kinases that mediate intracellular signaling pathways via SMAD proteins.[81] The complex then can translocate into the nucleus to alter gene expression.[81] TGF-βI and TGF-βII also stimulate the synthesis of Snail (SNAI1) and Slug (SNAI2), two transcription factors that have been shown to drive EMT by leading to the loss of E-cadherin expression.[82] TGF-β is also known to promote tumor invasion by increasing the expression of matrix metalloproteinases (MMPs), including MMP-1, MMP-3, MMP-9, and MMP-10.[81] In addition, TGF-β has been shown to promote the transition of stromal cells into cancer-associated fibroblasts (CAFs), which also play a prominent role in EMT and metastasis.[83]

Fibroblasts in the TME are capable of transforming into CAFs, which exhibit myofibroblastic features and express α–smooth muscle actin (α-SMA).[83,84] CAFs secrete a collection of cytokines, chemokines, and growth factors as well as inflammatory mediators and ECM proteins.[83] This characteristic collection of chemokines mediates the tumor-stromal cross-talk that enhances angiogenesis, lymphangiogenesis, and metastasis.[84,85] When compared with normal oral fibroblasts, CAFs secrete higher levels of activin A, a member of TGF-β family, to promote tumor cell proliferation and invasion.[83] CAFs produce high levels of TGF-βI and TGF-βII in only a subset of OSCC tumors that carry *TP53* and *CDKN2A* loss-of-function mutations.[86] In addition, CAFs affect the immune cells in the TME, specifically by acting on macrophages in the TME to promote an immunosuppressive environment.[87] Macrophages, known as tumor-associated macrophages (TAMs), are the most abundant immune cells in the TME.[87] TAMs exist in two functional phenotypes: M1 macrophages, which produce proinflammatory cytokines that lead to an antitumor effect; and M2 macrophages, which have an immunosuppressive function, stimulate angiogenesis, and enhance tumor cell invasion.[87,88] The specific inflammatory cytokines (eg, interleukin-6 and CXCL8) produced by CAFs enrich M2 population, which therefore allows for immunosuppression within the TME.[87]

Thus, through the TGF-β signaling pathway, OSCC cells can act on their microenvironment to promote cell proliferation, the production of MMPs to digest the basement membrane, and the transformation of oral fibroblasts into CAFs. These interactions further promote metastasis, local immunosuppression, and tumor invasion.

OMICS TECHNOLOGY IN UNDERSTANDING THE PATHOBIOLOGICAL MECHANISMS OF ORAL SQUAMOUS CELL CARCINOMA

To obtain the most optimal patient outcome, medical care strategies in cancer medicine include effective prevention, early detection, and diagnosis as well as efficacious treatment with minimal toxicities. In this post-genomics era, our understanding of cancer pathobiology has gradually transitioned from a morphology-based to a genetics-based system.[89] As discussed previously, OSCC is a complex genetic disease exhibiting tumor heterogeneity and tumor plasticity.[29] Medical care decisions need to be customized based on the unique genomic and proteomic features of each individual tumor. To address OSCC tumor heterogeneity and individual variations, current research uses omics technologies, such as genomics, transcriptomics, proteomics, and metabolomics, with the goal of identifying biomarkers based on tumor biopsies, circulating tumor cells, or body fluid (eg, saliva).[90] Omics technologies are high-throughput screening methodologies that can qualitatively and quantitatively analyze target molecules (eg, transcripts) in one experiment.[91] Unlike conventional cancer genetic research that addresses one or a few signaling pathways at a time, omics technologies provide a comprehensive and unbiased overview of the genome-scale or proteome-scale data sets.[91] With the aid of bioinformatics, an enormous amount of information is generated, and the complex, clinically meaningful effects can, therefore, be uncovered. The integration of omics technologies, bioinformatics, and conventional molecular biology has dramatically changed the landscape of cancer research and has a great impact on the understanding of the disease process.[92] Furthermore, with its improved accuracy and efficiency, omics technologies now have extended their role to molecular diagnostics and biomarker discovery.[91] The recent applications of omics technologies in investigating the pathobiological mechanisms of OSCC are reviewed.

Genomics in Oral Squamous Cell Carcinoma Research

Genomics-related technology includes whole-genome sequencing and whole-exome sequencing. There are multiple commercial platforms available for identifying gene mutations, SNPs, or copy number alterations.[91] The Cancer Genome Atlas (TCGA), launched in 2005, is a collaboration between the National Cancer Institute (NCI) and the National Human Genome Research Institute.[93] TCGA has generated comprehensive, multidimensional maps of key genomic changes in thirty-three types of cancer, including head and neck SCC.[93] The comprehensive genomic profiling has revealed two distinct subtypes of oral and oropharyngeal SCC: HPV-negative tumors, which typically arise in oral cavity proper and lips; and HPV-positive tumors, which mainly present in the oropharynx.[51,52,93] These two subtypes of SCC harbor distinct molecular alterations that correspond to their clinical behavior and patient prognosis.[93] Consistent with prior studies, the TCGA database revealed that a vast majority of HPV-negative OSCCs exhibit *TP53* loss-of-function mutations and *CDKN2A* inactivation.[93] In addition, integrated genomic analyses indicated a high level of heterogeneity in HPV-negative OSCC.[93] Novel mutations overlooked in the previous studies were discovered using whole-exome sequencing, a transcriptomics technique for sequencing all of the expressed genes in a genome (known as the exome).[51,52] Mutations in *NOTCH1* occurred in approximately 15% of cases, and mutations and focal copy-number alterations of *NOTCH2/3* were detected in the additional 11% of OSCC cases.[51,52]

The astonishing heterogeneity of OSCC illustrates how precision medicine can truly benefit patients and improve medical care. Further advancing from whole-exome sequencing to whole-genome sequencing, the PanCancer Analysis of Whole Genomes project (PCAWG) is now steered to reveal noncoding driver mutations, including alternative promoter usage, splicing, expression, editing, fusion, allele-specific expression, and nonsynonymous variants.[94] These noncoding transcripts, namely miRNAs and long noncoding RNAs (lncRNAs), demonstrate a tremendous potential for further clinical inquiries.[95,96]

Transcriptomics in Oral Squamous Cell Carcinoma Research

Extensive efforts have been distributed to characterize OSCC at the molecular level with transcriptomics technology.[97] To improve the therapeutic regimens for the managements of OSCC, reliable biomarkers are required to facilitate the prediction of clinical outcome and monitor treatment efficacy. When surveying a cohort of OSCC transcriptomes, dysregulation of multiple pathways (eg, mRNA processing, cytoskeletal organization, metabolic processes, cell cycle regulation, and apoptosis) was detected.[97] Similar to lung SCC, molecular characterization of OSCC has also been proposed.[98] Affected signaling pathways include dysregulation of the KEAP1/NFE2L2 oxidative stress pathway, differential utilization of the lineage markers SOX2 and TP63, and PIK3CA and EGFR mutations.[98] Clinically distinct behaviors are associated with different activation patterns of the EGFR pathway.[99] A molecular signature has also been proposed to predict the presence of lymph node metastases using the primary tumor at the time of diagnosis to assist in treatment planning for OSCC.[99,100] In addition, microarray data revealed the overexpression of BGH3, MMP9, and PDIA3 in more than 80% of OSCC tumors, suggesting the importance of ECM-cell receptor interactions in OSCC progression.[101] For potential clinical applications, these transcriptional signatures can be complementary in facilitating the formation of personalized therapeutic regimens in the management of OSCC.

Proteomics and Phospho-proteomics in Oral Squamous Cell Carcinoma Research

A landmark study in 2011 measuring the absolute mRNA and protein abundance and turnover by parallel metabolic pulse labeling revealed that cellular abundance of proteins is predominantly controlled by the level of translation.[102] Although mRNA and protein levels do correlate to a certain extent, genome-wide protein abundance is still a crucial parameter to understand cellular state and function. High-throughput analyses of both total and phosphorylated proteins allow for investigation of intracellular and secreted proteins in body fluid specimens (eg, serum, plasma, urine, and saliva).[103] Proteomic analysis, complemented with in situ hybridization or immunohistochemistry, has revealed altered expression at the protein level in cell metabolism, adhesion, motility, and signal transduction.[104-106] Studies have demonstrated promising results in distinguishing OSCC and normal samples by salivary or serum proteomics analyses with sensitivity and specificity as high as 80% to 90%.[106,107]

Metabolomics and Lipidomics in Oral Squamous Cell Carcinoma Research

Aided by mass spectrometry-based metabolomics analysis, metabolite profiling of tissue and body fluid specimens with the goal of biomarker discovery in OSCC research has revealed significant changes in energy metabolism pathways (eg, glycolysis and tricarboxylic acid cycle).[108] In the serum specimens from OSCC patients, the level of glycolytic metabolites (eg, glucose) are higher, with lower levels of certain amino acids (ie, valine, tyrosine, serine, and methionine).[109] On the contrary, such metabolite expression patterns are reversed in OSCC tumor tissues, suggesting the clinical implication of this signature panel as a screening tool.[109] Furthermore, OSCC cells can be subclassified into different groups based on their metabolic phenotypes (pyruvate, succinic acid, malic acid, citric acid, fumaric acid, and alphaketoglutaric acid) using high performance ion chromatography.[110] The clinical correlations discovered in these early studies, however, need to be validated by well-designed experiments. Lipids have also been identified as an important class of metabolites, and altered circulatory cholesterol levels have been linked to multiple cancer types.[111–113] It was reported that the levels of total lipids, cholesterol, and high-density lipoprotein were significantly lower in OSCC patients compared with healthy controls.[113,114] Although still primitive, these lipidomic data may suggest increased utilization by neoplastic cells for new membrane biogenesis and warrant further investigation.

With the rapid development of the omics tools discussed previously, these technologies will be collectively powerful with the potential to reveal molecular mechanisms and crucial signaling pathways driving the disease. In addition, these tools can be used to pinpoint novel therapeutic targets as well as nominate biomarkers that can be utilized in cancer diagnosis, prognosis prediction, and treatment surveillance.

FROM SCIENCE TO MEDICINE: THE INTEGRATION AND APPLICATION OF BIG DATA ON PERSONALIZED MANAGEMENTS OF ORAL CANCER

Based on the definition provided by the NCI, precision medicine, also known as personalized medicine, is "an approach to patient care that allows doctors to select treatments that are most likely to help patients based on a genetic understanding of their disease."[115] With the evolution of omics technologies, a large amount of information has been gained from the molecular profiling of OSCC tumors. Clinicians and scientists are expected to collaborate and translate these findings into medication targets for treating OSCC.[116] Typically, cancer-specific cell receptors or intracellular signaling molecules are targeted by either monoclonal antibodies (eg, cetuximab) or synthetic small molecules (eg, gefinitib).[22] Omics data addressing molecular changes alone, however, are insufficient to implement genomics-based precision medicine.[92] More importantly, we need to understand how these aberrant genes contribute to the tumor behaviors (eg, determinant of metastasis, response to a particular drug). It is known that omics data harbor a noisy mixture of cancer-causing mutations and bystander mutations.[117] Thus, in addition to generating cancer genomic data, more efforts should be directed to the identification and functional validation of the cancer-causing mutations.

After candidate mutation discovery by omics-scale methods, the next crucial step is to generate a clinically relevant hypothesis and design well-controlled experiments in tissue culture or animal models to validate the role of each candidate mutation in the cancer-related activities, such as invasiveness and interactions with the surrounding microenvironment.[118,119] In addition, it is critical to correlate experimental data with clinical presentations and confirm the expression of target mutations in human specimens by immunohistochemistry, fluorescence in situ hybridization (FISH), or gene expression microarray.[115] In the beginning of the biomarker discovery and drug design process, it is also important to characterize the biochemical and structural features of the target protein. Thus, we can screen based on the activity of compounds in a library, and then optimize its drug-like property and measure its potency, specificity, and pharmacokinetic characteristics. Initiatives by national and international consortia, such as the Cancer Therapy Evaluation Program organized by the NCI and International Cancer Genomics Consortium, coordinate resources and efforts to investigate comprehensive molecular profiling for multiple cancer types, as well as develop and assess novel targeted anticancer drugs and sponsor clinical trials.[120] Thus far, there are four large-scale head and neck cancer projects globally and in the United States.[120] Finally, ethical considerations derived from the medical advancement (eg, privacy, confidentiality, and potential possibility for discrimination) also need to be addressed.[120] Readers are referred to the published guidelines and recommendations for detailed regulations.[121]

SUMMARY

OSCC is a distinct subtype of head and neck SCC with traditional risk factors, such as tobacco, alcohol, and areca nut. These cancers are predominantly HPV negative and harbor *TP53* loss-of-function mutations. Although there are now highly sophisticated diagnostic systems, OSCCs are primarily treated with surgical excision and cervical lymph node dissection, both of which are associated with high morbidity and mortality. Prognosis remains dismal with an approximately 50% 5-year survival rate for advanced OSCC tumors. OSCCs are heterogeneous tumors with genetic and epigenetic aberrations, encompassing a wide range of oncogenic pathways (eg, PI3K-PTEN-AKT-mTOR). With the advent of genomic, proteomic, and metabolomic profiling, comprehensive biomarkers have been discovered that can identify tumors with greater invasive and metastatic potential. Investigation of new and currently identified biomarkers in the validation cohorts and multicenter clinical trials will further pave the way for developing truly personalized therapy for OSCC patients.

REFERENCES

1. Ferlay J, Soerjomataram I, Dikshit R, et al. Cancer incidence and mortality worldwide: sources, methods and major patterns in GLOBOCAN 2012. Int J Cancer 2015;136:E359–86.
2. Warnakulasuriya S. Living with oral cancer: epidemiology with particular reference to prevalence and life-style changes that influence survival. Oral Oncol 2010;46:407–10.
3. Siegel RL, Miller KD, Jemal A. Cancer statistics, 2016. CA Cancer J Clin 2016; 66:7–30.
4. Siegel R, Ma J, Zou Z, et al. Cancer statistics, 2014. CA Cancer J Clin 2014; 64(1):9–29.
5. Siegel R, Naishadham D, Jemal A. Cancer statistics, 2013. CA Cancer J Clin 2013;63:11–30.
6. Siegel R, Naishadham D, Jemal A. Cancer statistics, 2012. CA Cancer J Clin 2012;62:10–29.
7. Siegel R, Ward E, Brawley O, et al. Cancer statistics, 2011: the impact of eliminating socioeconomic and racial disparities on premature cancer deaths. CA Cancer J Clin 2011;61:212–36.
8. Jemal A, Siegel R, Xu J, et al. Cancer statistics, 2010. CA Cancer J Clin 2010;60: 277–300.
9. de Camargo Cancela M, de Souza DL, Curado MP. International incidence of oropharyngeal cancer: a population-based study. Oral Oncol 2012;48:484–90.
10. D'Souza G, Kreimer AR, Viscidi R, et al. Case-control study of human papillomavirus and oropharyngeal cancer. N Engl J Med 2007;356:1944–56.
11. Ang KK, Harris J, Wheeler R, et al. Human papillomavirus and survival of patients with oropharyngeal cancer. N Engl J Med 2010;363:24–35.
12. McBride KA, Ballinger ML, Killick E, et al. Li-Fraumeni syndrome: cancer risk assessment and clinical management. Nat Rev Clin Oncol 2014;11:260–71.
13. Romick-Rosendale LE, Lui VW, Grandis JR, et al. The Fanconi anemia pathway: repairing the link between DNA damage and squamous cell carcinoma. Mutat Res 2013;743-744:78–88.
14. Kutler DI, Auerbach AD, Satagopan J, et al. High incidence of head and neck squamous cell carcinoma in patients with Fanconi anemia. Arch Otolaryngol Head Neck Surg 2003;129:106–12.

15. Scully C, Langdon J, Evans J. Marathon of eponyms: 26 Zinsser-Engman-Cole syndrome (Dyskeratosis congenita). Oral Dis 2012;18:522–3.

16. Chen YK, Huang HC, Lin LM, et al. Primary oral squamous cell carcinoma: an analysis of 703 cases in southern Taiwan. Oral Oncol 1999;35:173–9.

17. Seiwert TY, Zuo Z, Keck MK, et al. Integrative and comparative genomic analysis of HPV-positive and HPV-negative head and neck squamous cell carcinomas. Clin Cancer Res 2015;21:632–41.

18. Bagan J, Sarrion G, Jimenez Y. Oral cancer: clinical features. Oral Oncol 2010; 46:414–7.

19. Warnakulasuriya S. Global epidemiology of oral and oropharyngeal cancer. Oral Oncol 2009;45:309–16.

20. Massano J, Regateiro FS, Januario G, et al. Oral squamous cell carcinoma: review of prognostic and predictive factors. Oral Surg Oral Med Oral Pathol Oral Radiol Endod 2006;102:67–76.

21. Goy J, Hall SF, Feldman-Stewart D, et al. Diagnostic delay and disease stage in head and neck cancer: a systematic review. Laryngoscope 2009;119:889–98.

22. Algazi AP, Grandis JR. Head and neck cancer in 2016: a watershed year for improvements in treatment? Nat Rev Clin Oncol 2017;14:76–8.

23. Schmitz S, Ang KK, Vermorken J, et al. Targeted therapies for squamous cell carcinoma of the head and neck: current knowledge and future directions. Cancer Treat Rev 2014;40:390–404.

24. Feller LL, Khammissa RR, Kramer BB, et al. Oral squamous cell carcinoma in relation to field precancerisation: pathobiology. Cancer Cell Int 2013;13:31.

25. Slaughter DP, Southwick HW, Smejkal W. Field cancerization in oral stratified squamous epithelium; clinical implications of multicentric origin. Cancer 1953; 6:963–8.

26. Simple M, Suresh A, Das D, et al. Cancer stem cells and field cancerization of oral squamous cell carcinoma. Oral Oncol 2015;51:643–51.

27. Braakhuis BJ, Tabor MP, Kummer JA, et al. A genetic explanation of Slaughter's concept of field cancerization: evidence and clinical implications. Cancer Res 2003;63:1727–30.

28. van Houten VM, Tabor MP, van den Brekel MW, et al. Mutated p53 as a molecular marker for the diagnosis of head and neck cancer. J Pathol 2002;198: 476–86.

29. Stucky A, Sedghizadeh PP, Mahabady S, et al. Single-cell genomic analysis of head and neck squamous cell carcinoma. Oncotarget 2017.

30. Sayed SI, Dwivedi RC, Katna R, et al. Implications of understanding cancer stem cell (CSC) biology in head and neck squamous cell cancer. Oral Oncol 2011;47:237–43.

31. Ehrensberger AH, Svejstrup JQ. Reprogramming chromatin. Crit Rev Biochem Mol Biol 2012;47:464–82.

32. Bjerkvig R, Tysnes BB, Aboody KS, et al. Opinion: the origin of the cancer stem cell: current controversies and new insights. Nat Rev Cancer 2005;5:899–904.

33. Prince ME, Sivanandan R, Kaczorowski A, et al. Identification of a subpopulation of cells with cancer stem cell properties in head and neck squamous cell carcinoma. Proc Natl Acad Sci U S A 2007;104:973–8.

34. Chen YS, Wu MJ, Huang CY, et al. CD133/Src axis mediates tumor initiating property and epithelial-mesenchymal transition of head and neck cancer. PLoS One 2011;6:e28053.

35. Clay MR, Tabor M, Owen JH, et al. Single-marker identification of head and neck squamous cell carcinoma cancer stem cells with aldehyde dehydrogenase. Head Neck 2010;32:1195–201.

36. Joshua B, Kaplan MJ, Doweck I, et al. Frequency of cells expressing CD44, a head and neck cancer stem cell marker: correlation with tumor aggressiveness. Head Neck 2012;34:42–9.

37. Weissman TA, Pan YA. Brainbow: new resources and emerging biological applications for multicolor genetic labeling and analysis. Genetics 2015;199: 293–306.

38. Driessens G, Beck B, Caauwe A, et al. Defining the mode of tumour growth by clonal analysis. Nature 2012;488:527–30.

39. Singh AK, Arya RK, Maheshwari S, et al. Tumor heterogeneity and cancer stem cell paradigm: updates in concept, controversies and clinical relevance. Int J Cancer 2015;136:1991–2000.

40. Schepers AG, Snippert HJ, Stange DE, et al. Lineage tracing reveals Lgr5+ stem cell activity in mouse intestinal adenomas. Science 2012;337:730–5.

41. Park IK, Morrison SJ, Clarke MF. Bmi1, stem cells, and senescence regulation. J Clin Invest 2004;113:175–9.

42. Tanaka T, Komai Y, Tokuyama Y, et al. Identification of stem cells that maintain and regenerate lingual keratinized epithelial cells. Nat Cell Biol 2013;15:511–8.

43. Tanaka T, Atsumi N, Nakamura N, et al. Bmi1-positive cells in the lingual epithelium could serve as cancer stem cells in tongue cancer. Sci Rep 2016;6:39386.

44. Chen D, Wu M, Li Y, et al. Targeting BMI1+ cancer stem cells overcomes chemoresistance and inhibits metastases in squamous cell carcinoma. Cell Stem Cell 2017;20:621–34.e6.

45. Argiris A, Karamouzis MV, Raben D, et al. Head and neck cancer. Lancet 2008; 371:1695–709.

46. Haddad RI, Shin DM. Recent advances in head and neck cancer. N Engl J Med 2008;359:1143–54.

47. Benhamou Y, Picco V, Pages G. The telomere proteins in tumorigenesis and clinical outcomes of oral squamous cell carcinoma. Oral Oncol 2016;57:46–53.

48. Leemans CR, Braakhuis BJ, Brakenhoff RH. The molecular biology of head and neck cancer. Nat Rev Cancer 2011;11:9–22.

49. Partridge M, Pateromichelakis S, Phillips E, et al. A case-control study confirms that microsatellite assay can identify patients at risk of developing oral squamous cell carcinoma within a field of cancerization. Cancer Res 2000;60: 3893–8.

50. Stadler ME, Patel MR, Couch ME, et al. Molecular biology of head and neck cancer: risks and pathways. Hematol Oncol Clin North Am 2008;22:1099–124, vii.

51. Agrawal N, Frederick MJ, Pickering CR, et al. Exome sequencing of head and neck squamous cell carcinoma reveals inactivating mutations in NOTCH1. Science 2011;333:1154–7.

52. Stransky N, Egloff AM, Tward AD, et al. The mutational landscape of head and neck squamous cell carcinoma. Science 2011;333:1157–60.

53. Opitz OG, Suliman Y, Hahn WC, et al. Cyclin D1 overexpression and p53 inactivation immortalize primary oral keratinocytes by a telomerase-independent mechanism. J Clin Invest 2001;108:725–32.

54. Chung CH, Guthrie VB, Masica DL, et al. Genomic alterations in head and neck squamous cell carcinoma determined by cancer gene-targeted sequencing. Ann Oncol 2015;26:1216–23.

55. Ongkeko WM, Altuna X, Weisman RA, et al. Expression of protein tyrosine kinases in head and neck squamous cell carcinomas. Am J Clin Pathol 2005; 124:71–6.
56. Choi S, Myers JN. Molecular pathogenesis of oral squamous cell carcinoma: implications for therapy. J Dent Res 2008;87:14–32.
57. Murugan AK, Hong NT, Fukui Y, et al. Oncogenic mutations of the PIK3CA gene in head and neck squamous cell carcinomas. Int J Oncol 2008;32:101–11.
58. Nicolas M, Wolfer A, Raj K, et al. Notch1 functions as a tumor suppressor in mouse skin. Nat Genet 2003;33:416–21.
59. Egger G, Liang G, Aparicio A, et al. Epigenetics in human disease and prospects for epigenetic therapy. Nature 2004;429:457–63.
60. Gasche JA, Goel A. Epigenetic mechanisms in oral carcinogenesis. Future Oncol 2012;8:1407–25.
61. Jithesh PV, Risk JM, Schache AG, et al. The epigenetic landscape of oral squamous cell carcinoma. Br J Cancer 2013;108:370–9.
62. Kulkarni V, Saranath D. Concurrent hypermethylation of multiple regulatory genes in chewing tobacco associated oral squamous cell carcinomas and adjacent normal tissues. Oral Oncol 2004;40:145–53.
63. Kato K, Hara A, Kuno T, et al. Aberrant promoter hypermethylation of p16 and MGMT genes in oral squamous cell carcinomas and the surrounding normal mucosa. J Cancer Res Clin Oncol 2006;132:735–43.
64. von Zeidler SV, Miracca EC, Nagai MA, et al. Hypermethylation of the p16 gene in normal oral mucosa of smokers. Int J Mol Med 2004;14:807–11.
65. Yoo CB, Jones PA. Epigenetic therapy of cancer: past, present and future. Nat Rev Drug Discov 2006;5:37–50.
66. Smith IM, Mydlarz WK, Mithani SK, et al. DNA global hypomethylation in squamous cell head and neck cancer associated with smoking, alcohol consumption and stage. Int J Cancer 2007;121:1724–8.
67. Kurdistani SK. Histone modifications in cancer biology and prognosis. Prog Drug Res 2011;67:91–106.
68. Easwaran H, Tsai HC, Baylin SB. Cancer epigenetics: tumor heterogeneity, plasticity of stem-like states, and drug resistance. Mol Cell 2014;54:716–27.
69. Webber LP, Wagner VP, Curra M, et al. Hypoacetylation of acetyl-histone H3 (H3K9ac) as marker of poor prognosis in oral cancer. Histopathology 2017; 71:278–86.
70. Koshizuka K, Hanazawa T, Fukumoto I, et al. The microRNA signatures: aberrantly expressed microRNAs in head and neck squamous cell carcinoma. J Hum Genet 2017;62:3–13.
71. Lu J, Getz G, Miska EA, et al. MicroRNA expression profiles classify human cancers. Nature 2005;435:834–8.
72. Lajer CB, Nielsen FC, Friis-Hansen L, et al. Different miRNA signatures of oral and pharyngeal squamous cell carcinomas: a prospective translational study. Br J Cancer 2011;104:830–40.
73. Lagos-Quintana M, Rauhut R, Lendeckel W, et al. Identification of novel genes coding for small expressed RNAs. Science 2001;294:853–8.
74. Bartel DP. MicroRNAs: genomics, biogenesis, mechanism, and function. Cell 2004;116:281–97.
75. Gorenchtein M, Poh CF, Saini R, et al. MicroRNAs in an oral cancer context - from basic biology to clinical utility. J Dent Res 2012;91:440–6.
76. Friedman RC, Farh KK, Burge CB, et al. Most mammalian mRNAs are conserved targets of microRNAs. Genome Res 2009;19:92–105.

77. Liu S, Liu L, Ye W, et al. High vimentin expression associated with lymph node metastasis and predicated a poor prognosis in oral squamous cell carcinoma. Sci Rep 2016;6:38834.

78. Ye X, Weinberg RA. Epithelial-mesenchymal plasticity: a central regulator of cancer progression. Trends Cell Biol 2015;25:675–86.

79. Yan TL, Wang M, Xu Z, et al. Up-regulation of syncytin-1 contributes to TNF-alpha-enhanced fusion between OSCC and HUVECs partly via Wnt/beta-catenin-dependent pathway. Sci Rep 2017;7:40983.

80. Curry JM, Sprandio J, Cognetti D, et al. Tumor microenvironment in head and neck squamous cell carcinoma. Semin Oncol 2014;41:217–34.

81. Hino M, Kamo M, Saito D, et al. Transforming growth factor-beta1 induces invasion ability of HSC-4 human oral squamous cell carcinoma cells through the Slug/Wnt-5b/MMP-10 signalling axis. J Biochem 2016;159:631–40.

82. Medici D, Hay ED, Olsen BR. Snail and slug promote epithelial-mesenchymal transition through beta-catenin-T-cell factor-4-dependent expression of transforming growth factor-beta3. Mol Biol Cell 2008;19:4875–87.

83. Bagordakis E, Sawazaki-Calone I, Macedo CC, et al. Secretome profiling of oral squamous cell carcinoma-associated fibroblasts reveals organization and disassembly of extracellular matrix and collagen metabolic process signatures. Tumour Biol 2016;37:9045–57.

84. Gandellini P, Andriani F, Merlino G, et al. Complexity in the tumour microenvironment: cancer associated fibroblast gene expression patterns identify both common and unique features of tumour-stroma crosstalk across cancer types. Semin Cancer Biol 2015;35:96–106.

85. Lin NN, Wang P, Zhao D, et al. Significance of oral cancer-associated fibroblasts in angiogenesis, lymphangiogenesis, and tumor invasion in oral squamous cell carcinoma. J Oral Pathol Med 2017;46:21–30.

86. Cirillo N, Hassona Y, Celentano A, et al. Cancer-associated fibroblasts regulate keratinocyte cell-cell adhesion via TGF-beta-dependent pathways in genotype-specific oral cancer. Carcinogenesis 2017;38:76–85.

87. Takahashi H, Sakakura K, Kudo T, et al. Cancer-associated fibroblasts promote an immunosuppressive microenvironment through the induction and accumulation of protumoral macrophages. Oncotarget 2017;8:8633–47.

88. Fujii N, Shomori K, Shiomi T, et al. Cancer-associated fibroblasts and CD163-positive macrophages in oral squamous cell carcinoma: their clinicopathological and prognostic significance. J Oral Pathol Med 2012;41:444–51.

89. Zhang X, Li L, Wei D, et al. Moving cancer diagnostics from bench to bedside. Trends Biotechnol 2007;25:166–73.

90. Wang X, Kaczor-Urbanowicz KE, Wong DT. Salivary biomarkers in cancer detection. Med Oncol 2017;34:7.

91. Kim DH, Kim YS, Son NI, et al. Recent omics technologies and their emerging applications for personalised medicine. IET Syst Biol 2017;11:87–98.

92. Chin L, Andersen JN, Futreal PA. Cancer genomics: from discovery science to personalized medicine. Nat Med 2011;17:297–303.

93. Cancer Genome Atlas Network. Comprehensive genomic characterization of head and neck squamous cell carcinomas. Nature 2015;517:576–82.

94. Stein LD, Knoppers BM, Campbell P, et al. Data analysis: create a cloud commons. Nature 2015;523:149–51.

95. Wiklund ED, Gao S, Hulf T, et al. MicroRNA alterations and associated aberrant DNA methylation patterns across multiple sample types in oral squamous cell carcinoma. PLoS One 2011;6:e27840.

96. Tang H, Wu Z, Zhang J, et al. Salivary lncRNA as a potential marker for oral squamous cell carcinoma diagnosis. Mol Med Rep 2013;7:761–6.
97. Severino P, Alvares AM, Michaluart P Jr, et al. Global gene expression profiling of oral cavity cancers suggests molecular heterogeneity within anatomic subsites. BMC Res Notes 2008;1:113.
98. Walter V, Yin X, Wilkerson MD, et al. Molecular subtypes in head and neck cancer exhibit distinct patterns of chromosomal gain and loss of canonical cancer genes. PLoS One 2013;8:e56823.
99. Chung CH, Parker JS, Karaca G, et al. Molecular classification of head and neck squamous cell carcinomas using patterns of gene expression. Cancer Cell 2004;5:489–500.
100. van Hooff SR, Leusink FK, Roepman P, et al. Validation of a gene expression signature for assessment of lymph node metastasis in oral squamous cell carcinoma. J Clin Oncol 2012;30:4104–10.
101. He Y, Shao F, Pi W, et al. Largescale transcriptomics analysis suggests overexpression of BGH3, MMP9 and PDIA3 in oral squamous cell carcinoma. PLoS One 2016;11:e0146530.
102. Schwanhausser B, Busse D, Li N, et al. Global quantification of mammalian gene expression control. Nature 2011;473:337–42.
103. Malik UU, Zarina S, Pennington SR. Oral squamous cell carcinoma: key clinical questions, biomarker discovery, and the role of proteomics. Arch Oral Biol 2016; 63:53–65.
104. Lo WY, Lai CC, Hua CH, et al. S100A8 is identified as a biomarker of HPV18-infected oral squamous cell carcinomas by suppression subtraction hybridization, clinical proteomics analysis, and immunohistochemistry staining. J Proteome Res 2007;6:2143–51.
105. Hu S, Wong DT. Oral cancer proteomics. Curr Opin Mol Ther 2007;9:467–76.
106. Schaaij-Visser TB, Brakenhoff RH, Leemans CR, et al. Protein biomarker discovery for head and neck cancer. J Proteomics 2010;73:1790–803.
107. Wadsworth JT, Somers KD, Stack BC Jr, et al. Identification of patients with head and neck cancer using serum protein profiles. Arch Otolaryngol Head Neck Surg 2004;130:98–104.
108. Wang J, Christison TT, Misuno K, et al. Metabolomic profiling of anionic metabolites in head and neck cancer cells by capillary ion chromatography with orbitrap mass spectrometry. Anal Chem 2014;86:5116–24.
109. Yonezawa K, Nishiumi S, Kitamoto-Matsuda J, et al. Serum and tissue metabolomics of head and neck cancer. Cancer Genomics Proteomics 2013;10:233–8.
110. Hu S, Wang J, Ji EH, et al. Targeted metabolomic analysis of head and neck cancer cells using high performance ion chromatography coupled with a Q exactive HF mass spectrometer. Anal Chem 2015;87:6371–9.
111. Tie G, Yan J, Khair L, et al. Hypercholesterolemia increases colorectal cancer incidence by reducing production of NKT and gammadelta T Cells from hematopoietic stem cells. Cancer Res 2017;77:2351–62.
112. Codini M, Cataldi S, Lazzarini A, et al. Why high cholesterol levels help hematological malignancies: role of nuclear lipid microdomains. Lipids Health Dis 2016; 15:4.
113. Acharya S, Rai P, Hallikeri K, et al. Serum lipid profile in oral squamous cell carcinoma: alterations and association with some clinicopathological parameters and tobacco use. Int J Oral Maxillofac Surg 2016;45:713–20.

114. Patel PS, Shah MH, Jha FP, et al. Alterations in plasma lipid profile patterns in head and neck cancer and oral precancerous conditions. Indian J Cancer 2004;41:25–31.
115. Tran B, Dancey JE, Kamel-Reid S, et al. Cancer genomics: technology, discovery, and translation. J Clin Oncol 2012;30:647–60.
116. Tonella L, Giannoccaro M, Alfieri S, et al. Gene expression signatures for head and neck cancer patient stratification: are results ready for clinical application? Curr Treat Options Oncol 2017;18:32.
117. Stratton MR, Campbell PJ, Futreal PA. The cancer genome. Nature 2009;458:719–24.
118. Mardis ER, Wilson RK. Cancer genome sequencing: a review. Hum Mol Genet 2009;18:R163–8.
119. Gonzalez-Angulo AM, Hennessy BT, Mills GB. Future of personalized medicine in oncology: a systems biology approach. J Clin Oncol 2010;28:2777–83.
120. Razzouk S. Translational genomics and head and neck cancer: toward precision medicine. Clin Genet 2014;86:412–21.
121. Fabsitz RR, McGuire A, Sharp RR, et al. Ethical and practical guidelines for reporting genetic research results to study participants: updated guidelines from a National Heart, Lung, and Blood Institute working group. Circ Cardiovasc Genet 2010;3:574–80.

Evaluation and Staging of Oral Cancer

Mel Mupparapu, DMD, MDS, Diplomate, ABOMR[a],*, Rabie M. Shanti, DMD, MD[b,c]

KEYWORDS

- Oral cancer • TNM classification • Tumor size • Lymph node metastases
- Squamous cell carcinoma • PET scan • MRI • CT scan

KEY POINTS

- In 1959, the American Joint Committee on Cancer and the International Union for Cancer Control, through a collaborative effort, developed cancer-specific staging systems.
- Since their inception more than 60 years ago, these worldwide cancer-specific staging benchmarks have been critically important in determining the extent of a cancer, guiding management, standardizing clinical trial participants, as well as in providing standardized systems in predicting prognosis.
- The tumor-node-metastasis (TNM) classification system has been outlined as having the following 6 objectives: (1) aid in treatment planning, (2) prognosis, (3) aid in the assessment of treatment results, (4) facilitate the exchange of information between institutions, (5) support cancer control activities, and (6) contribute to continuing investigation of human malignancies.

RATIONALE FOR CANCER STAGING

In 1959, the American Joint Committee on Cancer (AJCC) and the International Union for Cancer Control (UICC), through a collaborative effort, developed cancer-specific staging systems.[1] Since their inception more than 60 years ago, these worldwide cancer-specific staging benchmarks have been critically important in determining the extent of a cancer, guiding management, standardizing clinical trial participants and also in providing standardized systems in predicting prognosis.[1,2] The tumor-node-metastasis (TNM) classification system has been outlined as having the following 6 objectives: (1) aid in treatment planning, (2) prognosis, (3) aid in the assessment of treatment results, (4) facilitate the exchange of information between

Disclosure: The authors have no relevant disclosures.
[a] Oral Medicine, Department of Oral and Maxillofacial Surgery, Hospital of the University of Pennsylvania, Philadelphia, PA 19104, USA; [b] Department of Oral and Maxillofacial Surgery and Pharmacology, University of Pennsylvania School of Dental Medicine, Philadelphia, PA 19104, USA; [c] Department of Otorhinolaryngology/Head and Neck Surgery, Perelman School of Medicine University of Pennsylvania, Philadelphia, PA 19104, USA
* Corresponding author.
E-mail address: mmd@upenn.edu

Dent Clin N Am 62 (2018) 47–58
http://dx.doi.org/10.1016/j.cden.2017.08.003
0011-8532/18/© 2017 Elsevier Inc. All rights reserved.

institutions, (5) support cancer control activities, and (6) contribute to continuing investigation of human malignancies.[2–4]

Since the inception of a standardized TNM cancer staging system more than 60 years ago, various modifications have been made; however, the central theme of the AJCC and UICC staging system has been consistent. T refers to the extent of disease based on the size of the primary tumor and its local invasiveness. N refers to the presence or absence, size, and extent of regional lymph nodes. M refers to the presence or absence of distant metastasis. Currently, the TNM staging system that is in use for oral cancer was published in 2010 in the 7th edition of the manual published by the AJCC. In 2017, the 8th edition of this manual was released and its implementation will begin in January of 2018.[5]

TUMOR-NODE-METASTASIS STAGING OF ORAL CANCER

The first step in the staging process is identifying the histologic type of the lesion of interest. Squamous cell carcinoma (SCC), which comprises 90% of malignant neoplasms of the oral cavity and malignant neoplasms of the minor salivary glands within the oral cavity, share the same TNM staging system, whereas malignant melanoma has its own TNM staging system. Sarcomas of the oral cavity share the same staging system as sarcomas of the appendicular skeleton.

The staging process of a cancer is dynamic and modifiable as clinical and pathologic information is gathered during the workup and treatment process. For example, a patient who is being staged before surgery or a patient whose treatment is nonsurgical will have his or her cancer staged by using the clinical TNM (cTNM) system.[5] However, a patient who is being treated surgically will have his or her cancer staged based on the final surgical pathologic data and will have a separate pathologic TNM (pTNM) staging. The most recent staging, whether clinical or pathologic, will supersede previous TNM classifications in determining treatment recommendations and disease prognosis. Furthermore, aside from the "c" and "p" prefixes, the following prefixes are commonly used in cancer staging: "r" for recurrent tumor and "y" after radiation therapy and/or chemotherapy have been rendered. Of note, "r" and "y" prefixes are placed before "c" and "p" prefixes.

Tumor Classification

The tumor classification of a malignant neoplasm of the oral cavity describes the size of the primary tumor and its local invasiveness or extent. Tx denotes a situation when the primary tumor cannot be assessed. Tis within the oral cavity denotes a histologic diagnosis of SCC in situ irrespective of the size of the lesion; this T classification is only applicable to SCC. Therefore, Tis is not used for minor salivary gland neoplasms, sarcomas, or mucosal melanoma. However, when a diagnosis of invasive SCC has been rendered, T1, T2, and T3 classifications describe the primary lesion in its greatest surface dimension (**Fig. 1**). In the 7th edition of the AJCC staging system, T1 was for a lesion less than or equal to 2 cm, T2 denoted a lesion that was greater than 2 and less than or equal to 4 cm, and T3 corresponded to a lesion greater than 4. The 8th edition of the AJCC staging system will no longer solely depend on the greatest dimension of the surface of the lesion with regard to T1, T2, and T3 lesions.[5] The 8th edition of the AJCC staging system will incorporate depth of invasion (DOI), which will be defined by the pathologist as a measurement from the basement membrane relative to an area of intact squamous mucosa, which will be denoted as the horizon.[5] The distance from the horizon to the area of greatest invasion will serve as the measurement of DOI.[5] DOI is distinct from tumor thickness. The thickness of the tumor

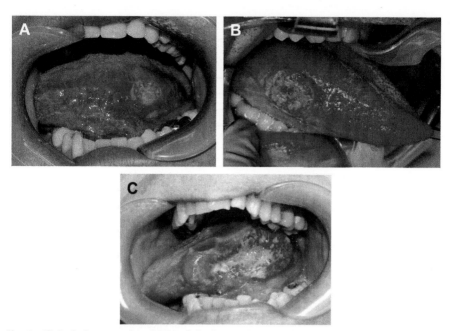

Fig. 1. Clinical photographs of SCC of the lateral border of the oral tongue. (*A*) T1 lesion, $\leq$2 cm. (*B*) T2 lesion, >2 and $\leq$4 cm. (*C*) T3 lesion, >4 cm.

is not incorporated into the TNM staging system for oral cavity SCC. The rationale for incorporating DOI for oral cavity SCC was based on strong evidence of DOI predicting risk for cervical lymph node metastasis, as well as prognosis, especially in patients with early stage oral SCC.[6–8] For example, a patient with a 3 cm SCC of the anterior floor of mouth with a DOI of 12 mm would have been staged as T2 based on the previous staging system; however, based on the 8th edition of the TNM staging system, the same lesion will be staged as T3.

Table 1 describes the T category for oral cavity SCC based on the 8th edition cancer-staging manual.[5] Therefore, in the TNM staging system, the T classifications of T1, T2, and T3 will depend on the greatest surface measurement of the lesion and the DOI that is obtained from initial biopsy or following surgical excision. The T4 category is currently subcategorized into T4a (moderately advanced local disease) and T4b (very advanced local disease), and describes the local invasiveness of the primary tumor. The T4a and T4b categories do not consider the surface dimensions of the lesion or the DOI. T4a category is applied to oral cavity SCC that invade adjacent structures, such as overlying skin, cortical bone of the mandible or maxilla, and/or maxillary sinus. Of note, invasion of the alveolar bone of the maxilla or mandible or tooth structure does not upstage a lesion to T4a (**Fig. 2**A, B), instead, it must be cortical bone invasion (see **Fig. 2**C). For SCC of the lip, the T4a category is applied to lesions that invade through the cortical bone of the mandible or maxilla and lesions that invade the inferior alveolar nerve, as well as the floor of mouth or the skin of the face (ie, nose, chin).[5] Previously, invasion of the extrinsic muscles of the tongue would upstage a cancer to T4a; however, in the 8th edition of the staging manual, invasion of any of the extrinsic muscles of the tongue is not considered in the staging process. T4b is applied to lesions that invade the masticator space, skull base, pterygoid plates, and/or encases the carotid artery (**Fig. 3**). As previously mentioned, the same TNM staging system is applied to SCC and minor salivary gland malignant

Table 1
Tumor category for non–human papilloma virus–associated (p16 negative) oral squamous cell carcinoma, 8th edition cancer staging manual

T Category	Tumor Size	Additional Criteria
TX	Not applicable	Primary tumor cannot be assessed
Tis	Not applicable	Carcinoma in situ
T1	≤2 cm, ≤5 mm DOI	No additional criteria
T2	≤2 cm, DOI ≥5 mm, and ≤10 mm or tumor ≥2 cm but ≤4 cm and DOI ≤10 mm	No additional criteria
T3	≥4 cm or any tumor >10 mm DOI	No additional criteria
T4	Not applicable	Moderate to advanced local disease
T4a	Not applicable	Oral cavity, lip, chin, or nose tumor invading cortical bone or involving inferior alveolar nerve, floor of the mouth, facial skin, bones of mandible, or maxilla affecting basal bone
T4b	Not applicable	Advanced local disease in which tumor invades masticator space, pterygoid plates, or skull base, and may or may not encase internal carotid artery

Adapted from Lydiatt WM, Patel SG, O'Sullivan B, et al. Head and Neck cancers—major changes in the American Joint Committee on Cancer eighth edition cancer staging manual. CA Cancer J Clin 2017;67:122–37; with permission.

neoplasms of the oral cavity. Malignant neoplasms of the minor salivary glands are staged based on their anatomic site of origin, and malignant neoplasms of the major (submandibular, sublingual, and parotid) salivary glands share the same TNM staging system.

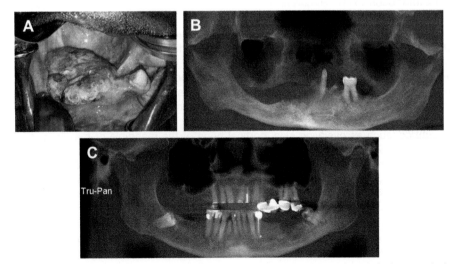

Fig. 2. (*A*) Clinical photograph of a T3 gingival SCC. (*B*) Panoramic radiograph showing lack of radiographic of invasion of the basal bone of the mandible, thus lesion was not upstaged to T4a. (*C*) Radiographic evidence of cortical bone invasion of the left body of the mandible.

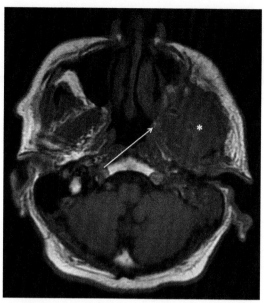

Fig. 3. T1W contrast-enhanced axial MRI of a recurrent SCC (*asterisk*) invading the left pterygoid plate (*arrow*), as well as the masticator space, skull base, and encasing the internal carotid artery (ICA), staging the tumor as T4b.

Table 2 describes the clinical and pathologic T stages (0–4) for human papilloma virus (HPV)-associated oropharyngeal cancer, 8th edition of the AJCC staging manual,[5] and is followed by a detailed description of each component of the TNM system for HPV-associated SCC of the oropharynx.

Mucosal melanoma has its own distinct T criteria. Tx similar to SCC denoted a situation in which the primary tumor cannot be assessed. T1 and T2 categories do not exist for mucosal melanoma. T3 refers to a mucosal melanoma that is limited to the mucosa. T4a refers to a lesion that invades the deep tissues (ie, overlying skin, muscles, bone, and cartilage). T4b refers to a lesion that invades the masticator space, prevertebral space, mediastinal structures, carotid artery, brain, dura, skull base,

Table 2	
Clinical and pathologic tumor category for human papilloma virus–associated (p16 positive) oropharyngeal cancer, 8th edition AJCC staging manual	
T Category	**Tumor Size and/or Additional Information**
T0	No identifiable primary lesion
T1	≤2 cm in greatest dimension
T2	2–4 cm in greatest dimension
T3	>4 cm in greatest dimension
T4	Moderately advanced local disease; tumor invading larynx, tongue muscle, medial pterygoid, hard palate, or mandible and beyond Mere mucosal invasion of lingual surface of epiglottis from primary tumors of tongue base and vallecula does not represent laryngeal invasion

Adapted from Lydiatt WM, Patel SG, O'Sullivan B, et al. Head and Neck cancers—major changes in the American Joint Committee on Cancer eighth edition cancer staging manual. CA Cancer J Clin 2017;67:122–37; with permission.

and lower cranial nerves (CNs), such as glossopharyngeal nerve (CN IX), vagus nerve (CN X), spinal accessory nerve (CN XI), and the hypoglossal nerve (CN XII).

Regional Lymph Nodes Classification

The lymph nodes of the neck serve as the first site of metastasis of oral SCC and all minor salivary gland cancers (excluding adenoid cystic carcinoma) and lymph node

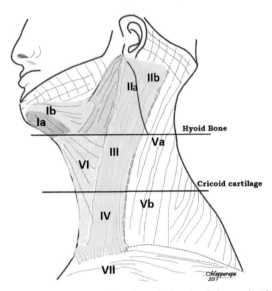

Fig. 4. Diagrammatic representation of lymph node levels of the neck. The hyoid bone and cricoid cartilage levels, crucial for identification of levels, are represented by horizontal lines. Level I nodes are below the mylohyoid muscle and above the lower margin of hyoid bone, as well as anterior and posterior borders of submandibular glands. Level Ia are submental nodes between the 2 anterior bellies of digastric. Level Ib indicate submandibular nodes that are posterolateral to the anterior belly of digastric. Level II nodes are internal jugular vein (IJV) or deep cervical chain, base of the skull to the carotid bifurcation, anterior to the posterior border of sternocleidomastoid (SCM) muscle, and posterior to the posterior border of the submandibular glands. Level IIa is inseparable from IJV. These are identified anterior (medial) to the vertical plane defined by CN XI. Level IIb is a fat plane separating the nodes and the vein. These are identified posterior (lateral) to the vertical plane defined by the CN XI. Level III nodes are IJV, lower margins of hyoid to lower margins of cricoid, anterior to the posterior border of SCM, and lateral to the medial margin of common carotid artery (CCA) and ICA. Level IV nodes are deep cervical (IJV) chain, lower margin of cricoid to clavicle, lateral to medial margin of CCA, and anterior and medial to an oblique line drawn through the posterior edge of SCM and the posterior edge of the anterior scalene muscle. Level V nodes are posterior triangle (spinal accessory) nodes that are subdivided. Va is the superior half, posterior to levels II and III from base of the skull and inferior border of cricoid. Vb is the inferior half, posterior to level IV (inferior border or cricoid and the level of clavicles). Level VI encompasses the pretracheal and prelaryngeal lymph nodes, anterior to the visceral space and from the inferior margin of hyoid bone to the manubrium. Level VII includes the superior mediastinal lymph nodes, as well as between CCAs, below the superior aspect of manubrium to level of the brachiocephalic vein. Predominance of certain levels was seen for each primary site. Levels I, II, and III were at highest risk for metastasis from cancer of the oral cavity. Levels II, III, and IV were at highest risk for metastasis from carcinomas of the oropharynx, hypopharynx, and larynx. (*Legend adapted from* Shah JP. Patterns of cervical lymph node metastasis from squamous carcinomas of the upper aerodigestive tract. Am J Surg 1990;160:405–9; with permission.)

groups in the neck are described by levels I to VII (**Fig. 4**). The presence of lymph node metastasis is considered the most important prognostic factor for SCC of the oral cavity, as well as all other head and neck subsites.[9] Lymph node metastasis is known to occur in 40% of cases of oral cavity SCC; however, 15% to 34% of these cases will have occult cervical nodal metastasis, which are deposits of tumor that are not apparent on clinical or radiographic assessment based on criteria of metastatic lymphadenopathy; however, cancer cells are identified on histologic analysis of a lymph nodes.[10] The absence or presence of lymph node metastasis in oral cavity SCC and minor salivary glands of the oral cavity is staged based on the criteria listed in **Table 3**.

Of note, a patient who has had surgical excision of their primary tumor and did not undergo a neck dissection will have their cancer staged as pT_NxM_. Similarly, a patient who had undergone a neck dissection and has not undergone resection of their primary tumor will be initially staged as pTxN_M_. Similar to what occurred with the T classification in incorporating DOI, the 8th edition of the staging manual will incorporate extracapsular extension (ECE) into the N category. ECE is defined by tumor invading beyond the lymph node capsule into the perinodal tissues (**Fig. 5**).[11]

An example of the staging process is highlighted in the following case of a 53-year-old woman who has never smoked with a 2.0 cm biopsy-proven SCC of the lateral border of the right oral tongue (see **Fig. 1**B) with a single ipsilateral level IIa lymph node measuring 2.2 in greatest transverse dimension (**Fig. 6**). PET–computed tomography (CT) did not identify any additional fluorodeoxyglucose (FDG)-avid lymph nodes and distant sites of FDG-avid metastatic disease were noted. The patient's clinical staging is cT2N1M0. **Fig. 7** denotes the clinical appearance of the aforementioned level IIa lymph node within the neck dissection packet.

Table 3
Regional lymph nodes pathologic category criteria for non–human papilloma virus–associated oropharyngeal cancer effective as of 2018

Node Category	Node Criteria
NX	Regional lymph nodes cannot be assessed
N0	No regional lymphadenopathy
N1	Metastases in a single ipsilateral lymph node ≤3 cm and ENE negative (–ve)
N2	Ipsilateral node ≤3 cm, ENE positive (+ve) 3–6 cm with ENE –ve Multiple ipsilateral metastatic lymph nodes none >6 cm and ENE –ve Metastatic bilateral or contralateral nodes <6 cm, ENE –ve
N2a	Ipsilateral single metastatic node ≤3 cm, ENE +ve Ipsilateral single metastatic node ≥3 cm but ≤6 cm, ENE –ve
N2b	Metastatic multiple ipsilateral nodes ≤6 cm, ENE –ve
N2c	Metastatic bilateral or contralateral lymph nodes ≤6 cm, ENE –ve
N3	Metastatic lymph nodes ≥6 cm, ENE –ve; metastatic single ipsilateral lymph node ≥3 cm, ENE +ve; metastatic multiple ipsilateral, contralateral or bilateral lymph nodes, ENE +ve
N3a	Metastatic lymph node ≥6 cm, ENE +ve
N3b	Metastatic single lymph node ≥3 cm, ENE +ve or metastatic multiple ipsilateral, bi or contralateral lymph nodes, ENE +ve

Abbreviation: ENE, extranodal extension.
Adapted from Lydiatt WM, Patel SG, O'Sullivan B, et al. Head and Neck cancers—major changes in the American Joint Committee on Cancer eighth edition cancer staging manual. CA Cancer J Clin 2017;67:122–37; with permission.

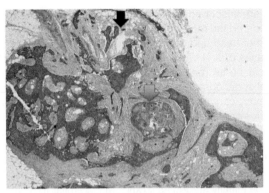

Fig. 5. Photomicrograph depicting the entire lymph node being replaced by the metastatic tumor with ECE in to the adjacent fat without any evidence of lymphoid remnants. Area where the lymph node is replaced by tumor (*blue arrow*). The tumor in the extranodal adipose tissue (*black arrow*). Hematoxylin-eosin stain (H&E × 20).

Distant Metastasis Classification

Distant metastasis is associated with high mortality, leading to a patient's death within 3 to 6 months of the diagnosis of distant metastatic disease.[12] The incidence of distant metastasis for oral cavity SCC has been reported to occur in 10% to 18% of patients at time of initial diagnosis.[13,14] Advanced T and N classifications are highly predictive for the presence of distant metastatic disease. Distant metastatic disease is most commonly identified by imaging studies (ie, PET-CT, CT, chest radiograph) and

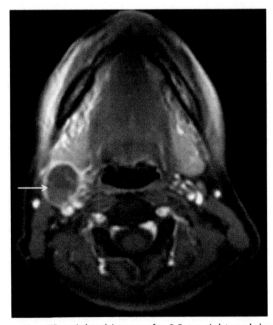

Fig. 6. Axial cross-section T2-weighted image of a 2.2 cm right neck level IIa lymph node (*arrow*).

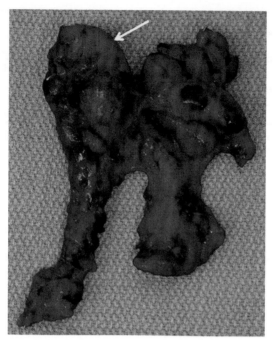

Fig. 7. Photograph of a neck dissection packet depicting the lymph node (*arrow*) in **Fig. 6**.

indirect blood tests (ie, liver function test). The details of the M classification system are described in **Table 4**.

The Mx designation is used until full workup for determining the presence or absence of distant metastasis has been performed. For instance, a patient who has had a PET-CT can have a designation of M0 (absence of distant metastasis) or M1 (presence of distant metastasis). However, a patient who only has a liver function test panel and no chest CT has a designation of Mx.

EVALUATION OF ORAL CANCER
Clinical Assessment

To properly stage a cancer, one must begin with an appropriate physical examination of the patient's head and neck, a thorough radiographic examination, and establishing a histologic diagnosis. This will involve measuring the size of the lesion in all its dimensions, palpating the depth of the lesion, and identifying any other lesions. A complete assessment of the patient will also involve palpating the right and left sides of the neck to clinically assess for lymphadenopathy. Palpable lymph nodes are staged per the aforementioned N classification system (**Fig. 8**). At times, the entirety of the lesion cannot be assessed based on in-office transoral examination due to gagging reflex or physical limitation in seeing the entirety of the lesion. In these cases, the patient is evaluated in the operating room via a direct laryngoscopy technique that incorporates the use of rigid and flexible cameras, and rigid metallic retractors or laryngoscopes (**Fig. 9**).

Radiographic Assessment

Imaging plays a significant role in the assessment of the primary site, regional lymph nodes, and distant structures to establish the clinical staging of a cancer. Oral and

Table 4
Distant metastasis classification system

Metastasis Category	Metastasis Criteria
Mx	Metastasis not determined Awaiting CT or PET examinations
M0	Distant metastasis not identified
M1	Distant metastasis identified

From Lydiatt WM, Patel SG, O'Sullivan B, et al. Head and Neck cancers—major changes in the American Joint Committee on Cancer eighth edition cancer staging manual. CA Cancer J Clin 2017;67:122–37; with permission.

oropharyngeal cancer spreads in 3 common ways. The cancer may spread by direct extension over mucosal surfaces, muscle, and bone; via lymphatic drainage pathways; or by extension along neurovascular bundles. For accurate staging of the cancer, evaluation of these 3 routes of spread is important.[15] In general, oral cavity and oropharyngeal SCCs can be visually inspected for the evaluation of mucosal spread. Superficial mucosal lesions are not often radiographically noted. The overall extent of the tumor can be often underestimated via physical examination alone because submucosal spread and direct invasion of the adjacent tissues cannot be assessed. The type of imaging acquired in the evaluation of an oral cancer depends on several factors, including the location of the lesion, stage of lesion, and practitioner or institutional preference. For example, it is common to obtain a panoramic radiograph in the initial assessment of a patient with oral cancer in preparation for surgery

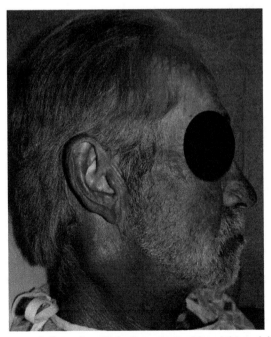

Fig. 8. Clinical photograph (lateral profile) of a patient with a right neck level IIa metastatic lymph node.

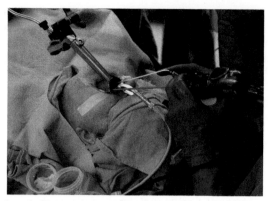

Fig. 9. Intraoperative photograph of rigid laryngoscopy and endoscope in place to assess the larynx, hypopharynx, and oropharynx for synchronous cancerous or precancerous lesions.

and/or radiation therapy to assess the health of the dentition and determination of cortical erosions. Furthermore, it is standard practice to obtain cross-sectional imaging to assess the primary site and regional cervical lymph nodes. The most common studies are MRI of the neck with intravenous (IV) contrast or CT of the neck with IV contrast. Subtle cortical erosions are detected with CT and the extent of marrow involvement is perhaps better assessed with MRI. To assess for distant metastasis, PET-CT has become the clinical imaging strategy of choice due to its higher detection rate of distant metastasis in comparison with other imaging modalities.[13]

SUMMARY

The staging of oral cancer using the TNM staging system allows for universally accepted standardization of a format that allows for communication between providers involved in the care of patients with cancer and in providing treatment recommendations. Furthermore, as more is learned about this disease process, the staging system must be dynamic to allow for incorporating and/or eliminating staging criteria, as evidenced by the new TNM staging system.

REFERENCES

1. Chavez-MacGregor M, Mittendorf EA, Clarke CA, et al. Incorporating tumor characteristics to the American Joint Committee on Cancer Breast Cancer Staging System. Oncologist 2017. [Epub ahead of print].
2. Gospodarowicz MK, Miller D, Groome PA, et al. The process for continuous improvement of the TNM classification. Cancer 2004;100:1–5.
3. Webber C, Gospodarowicz M, Sobin LH, et al. Improving the TNM classification: findings from a 10-year continuous literature review. Int J Cancer 2014;135: 371–8.
4. Sobin LH. TNM: principles, history, and relation to other prognostic factors. Cancer 2001;91(8 suppl):1589–92.
5. Lydiatt WM, Patel SG, O'Sullivan B, et al. Head and Neck cancers—major changes in the American Joint Committee on cancer eighth edition cancer staging manual. CA Cancer J Clin 2017;67:122–37.

6. Hori Y, Kubota A, Yokose T, et al. Predictive significance of tumor depth and budding for late lymph node metastases in patients with clinical n0 early oral tongue carcinoma. Head Neck Pathol 2017. [Epub ahead of print].

7. Mitani S, Tomioka T, Hayashi R, et al. Anatomic invasive depth predicts delayed cervical lymph node metastasis of tongue squamous cell carcinoma. Am J Surg Pathol 2016;40:934–42.

8. D'Cruz AK, Vaish R, Kapre N, et al. Head, neck disease management g: elective versus therapeutic neck dissection in node-negative oral cancer. N Engl J Med 2015;373:521–9.

9. Friedman M, Lim JW, Dickey W, et al. Quantification of lymph nodes in selective neck dissection. Laryngoscope 1999;109:368–70.

10. Noguti J, De Moura CF, De Jesus GP, et al. Metastasis from oral cancer: an overview. Cancer Genomics Proteomics 2012;9:329–35.

11. Lewis JS Jr, Tarabishy Y, Luo J, et al. Inter- and intra-observer variability in the classification of extracapsular extension in p16 positive oropharyngeal squamous cell carcinoma nodal metastases. Oral Oncol 2015;51:985–90.

12. Chen TC, Hsu CW, Lou PJ, et al. The clinical predictive factors for subsequent distant metastasis in patients with locoregionally advanced oral squamous cell carcinoma. Oral Oncol 2013;49:367–73.

13. Senft A, de Bree R, Hoekstra OS, et al. Screening for distant metastases in head and neck cancer patients by chest CT or whole body FDG-PET: a prospective multicenter trial. Radiother Oncol 2008;87:221–9.

14. Rohde M, Nielsen AL, Johansen J, et al. Head-to-head comparison of chest x-ray/head and neck MRI, chest CT/head and neck MRI, and 18F-FDG-PET/CT for detection of distant metastases and synchronous cancer in oral, pharyngeal, and laryngeal Cancer. J Nucl Med 2017. [Epub ahead of print].

15. Mukherji SK, Castelijns J, Castillo M. Squamous cell carcinoma of the oropharynx and oral cavity: how imaging makes a difference. Semin Ultrasound CT MR 1998; 19:463–75.

Adjunctive Diagnostic Techniques for Oral and Oropharyngeal Cancer Discovery

Michaell A. Huber, DDS

KEYWORDS

- Squamous cell carcinoma • Conventional oral examination • Biopsy
- Adjunctive aids

KEY POINTS

- The most important prognostic factor in predicting the outcome of oral and oropharyngeal cancer (OPC) is the stage at diagnosis.
- The accomplishment of the conventional oral examination consists of a disciplined visual and tactile assessment of accessible head and neck structures.
- Any suspicious or equivocal lesion should be referred for further assessment or undergo biopsy; innocuous lesions should be reevaluated within 4 weeks and referred for further assessment.
- Evidence supporting the use of adjunctive devices to improve the general practitioner's ability to screen for and identify OPCs and oral premalignant lesions remains low.

INTRODUCTION

For 2017, an estimated 49,670 individuals (35,720 men and 13,950 women) were diagnosed with oral and oropharyngeal cancer (OPC) in the United States.[1] The most important prognostic factor in predicting the outcome of OPC is the stage at which it is diagnosed.[2–6] The growth rates for OPC vary dramatically, with tumor volume doubling times ranging from 26 to 256 days, with a mean of about 3 months.[7,8] It has been clearly demonstrated that the discovery of OPC by the oral health care provider (OHP) during the accomplishment of a non–symptom-driven oral examination is associated with an earlier stage diagnosis and improved patient outcomes, when compared with the discovery of OPC by a physician performing a symptom-driven examination.[9] Unfortunately, only 30% of patients diagnosed with OPC in 2017 presented with localized disease.[1] Although the overall 5-year survival rates for OPC have gradually improved from 52.8% to 66.2% over the last 4 decades,[10] the

Disclosure: None.
Department of Comprehensive Dentistry, UT Health San Antonio School of Dentistry, 7703 Floyd Curl Drive (Mail Code 7919), San Antonio, TX 78229, USA
E-mail address: huberm@uthscsa.edu

Dent Clin N Am 62 (2018) 59–75
http://dx.doi.org/10.1016/j.cden.2017.08.004
0011-8532/18/© 2017 Elsevier Inc. All rights reserved.

OHP's success in identifying OPCs at an early stage remains a challenge. The purpose of this article is to discuss the current standard for identifying OPCs and the current status of novel adjunctive approaches being marketed to the dental profession.

DELAYS IN DISCOVERY OF ORAL AND OROPHARYNGEAL CANCER

In addressing the delay in the discovery of OPC, 2 distinct categories that have been traditionally discussed are patient delay and professional delay.[5,6,11] Patient delay is the time delay between the patient's first awareness of a change and his or her presentation to a health care provider. The parameters of professional delay are variable and represent the time delay between the first presentation to the health care provider and a specific endpoint (eg, biopsy, referral to a specialist, initiation of therapy).[5,6]

Patient delay represents the single most important factor underlying the delayed discovery of OPC.[5] In a retrospective study of 646 patients over a 19-year period, Friedrich[12] reported the most commonly noted signs and symptoms driving the patient to seek evaluation were localized swelling (n = 327), pain (n = 200), and mucosal changes (n = 167). The percentages for those who sought medical care for localized swelling, pain, or mucosal changes within 1 month were 46.4%, 43.0%, 41.4%, respectively. More problematic was finding that 15.2% of those with a localized swelling, 16.0% of those in pain, and 17.4% of those with a mucosal change waited more than 6 months before seeking medical care. Peacock and associates[13] prospectively studied a cohort of 50 patients with oral cancer and determined the mean time gap between the first symptom and the initial visit to a health care professional was 105 days (range, 0–730).

To date, there is no clear consensus to adequately explain the issue of patient delay.[14,15] Proposed reasons include patient psychosocial factors, health-related behaviors, socioeconomic status, education level, and health care access or availability.[5,15,16] Regardless of the ambiguity as to why, it is well-known that the public's interaction with the oral health care profession is low. In a recent Gallup report of interviews conducted during 2008 (n = 354,645) and 2013 (n = 178,072), only 64.7% of participants reported visiting a dentist within the past year.[17] Furthermore, patients at increased risk for OPC (eg, age >40 years, male gender, alcohol drinkers, tobacco smokers, low fruit and vegetable intake) are more likely to avoid routine dental care.[18] Clearly, concerted efforts to improve public awareness of OPC and the importance of early diagnosis are essential to addressing the issue of patient delay.[11,12,16,19] In this regard, the oral health care professional has a professional obligation to lead the conversation with his or her patient regarding the risk factors, signs, and symptoms of OPC.

The most relevant form of professional delay is the time from first encounter with the health care system to the initiation of definitive treatment. Ideally, any patient with an oral potentially malignant lesion (OPML) is afforded a prompt diagnosis and initiation of therapy. In the aforementioned study by Peacock and colleagues,[13] the mean professional delay from initial encounter to initiation of treatment was 101 days. Using an ideal goal of 30 days from first visit to the specialist to initiation of definitive treatment, Brouha et al[20] determined that the goal was met for only 41% of 134 patients with OPC.[20] Thus, although most patients diagnosed with cancer desire to initiate therapy immediately, many experience significant delays.[20,21]

CURRENT STANDARD FOR IDENTIFYING AND DIAGNOSING ORAL AND OROPHARYNGEAL CANCER

In daily practice, when the oral health care professional examines a patient, the clinician looks for any abnormality, not just OPC.[22] OPC screening does not exist as an isolated event, but as an integral component of the opportunistic comprehensive hard and soft tissue examination afforded all patients. The conventional oral examination (COE), which entails the use of appropriate lighting to accomplish a thorough visual and tactile assessment of accessible extraoral and intraoral tissues, remains the foundation upon which lesions are discovered.[4] A recently published consensus document identified the essential elements of such an examination for all patients, regardless of risk, and is summarized in **Table 1**.[2]

When accomplished in a disciplined manner, the sensitivity and specificity of oral inspection is 94% and 99%, respectively.[23] However, the ability to visually discriminate whether a given discovered lesion is benign or malignant is poor and the "gold standard" by which any equivocal lesion is diagnosed is the tissue biopsy.[11,24,25] Any suspicious or equivocal lesion should be referred for further assessment or undergo biopsy, whereas innocuous lesions should be reevaluated within 4 weeks and referred for further assessment or undergo biopsy if still present. Unfortunately, there is concern that not all OHPs accomplish a thorough COE on their patients, thus missing opportunities to diagnose OPCs at their earliest stage.[4,26,27] In a survey assessing the efficacy of continuing education efforts to address OPC early detection, Silverman and colleagues[4] determined that OHP awareness of what steps constituted a proper OPC screening examination improved from 82.6% at baseline to 92.7% at 6 months after training. The reported compliance in accomplishing a neck palpation after the training only improved from 60% to 69.1%, illustrating the continual need to improve clinician performance in accomplishing the extraoral component of the head and neck examination.

Table 1	
Elements of a proper conventional oral examination	
Extraoral examination	Perioral and intraoral examination
Visual inspection of the face, head, and neck to detect	Visual inspection[b] and manual palpation
Asymmetry	Lips, including external commissures[c]
Swelling	Labial mucosa and vestibule
Discoloration	Buccal mucosa, sulcus, and internal commissures
Ulceration	Gingiva and alveolar ridge
Skin changes[a]	Anterior tongue (up to circumvallate)
Manual palpation of	Dorsum
Nodes	Lateral
Preauricular lymph nodes	Ventral
Posterior auricular lymph nodes	Base of the tongue (including lingual tonsils)
Submandibular lymph nodes	Floor of the mouth
Anterior deep cervical lymph nodes	Palate
Posterior deep cervical lymph nodes	Hard palate
Neck	Soft palate
	Retromolar trigone area
	Visual inspection[c]
	Palatine tonsils
	Posterior pharyngeal wall

[a] Crusts, fissuring, growths.
[b] Visual inspection to detect asymmetry, swelling, discoloration, ulceration, or skin changes.
[c] Color, texture and surface abnormality.
Adapted from Li L, Morse DE, Katz RV. What constitutes a proper routine oral cancer examination for patients at low risk? Findings from a Delphi survey. Oral Surg Oral Med Oral Pathol Oral Radiol 2013;116:e379–86; with permission.

ADJUNCTIVE DIAGNOSTIC TECHNOLOGIES

One response to address this perceived diagnostic tardiness has been the development and marketing of numerous novel adjunctive technologies with the goal of improving the OHP's ability to screen for and identify OPCs and OPMLs at their earliest presentation.[28–42] They are all marketed as aids for the clinician to use in addition to, not in lieu of, the accomplishment of the COE and are often aggressively promoted as advanced and necessary products. Currently marketed adjuncts to identify OPCs and OPMLs are listed in **Tables 2** and **3**. Some of the adjuncts are marketed as "discovery or screening" enhancements to the COE, and others are marketed as case assessment utilities to further assess a visually identified lesion. Some are marketed as both.

Lingen and colleagues[25] have proposed objective criteria against which emerging adjunctive technologies may be objectively assessed (**Box 1**). Given the low prevalence of OPC, clinicians should pay attention to an adjunctive technology's sensitivity and specificity when it is promoted as a discovery tool to be used as an enhancement to the COE. None of the adjunctive test are diagnostic for oral cancer.

ROLE OF THE US FOOD AND DRUG ADMINISTRATION IN REGULATING ADJUNCTIVE TECHNOLOGIES

The OralCDx Brush Test (CDx Diagnostics, Suffern, NY), CytID (Forward Science, Houston, TX), and MOP cytology component (PCG Molecular, Cumming, GA) are all essentially laboratory processes, in which a cytology specimen is submitted for final review by a pathologist. As such, they are not devices requiring clearance by the US Food and Drug Administration (FDA).[43] Some of the adjunctive test companies will note they are certified under the Clinical Laboratory Improvement Amendments (CLIA) program.[44] However, CLIA certification simply means the laboratory is meeting certain performance standards to ensure their results are accurate and reliable. CLIA certification does not address the clinical validity or predictive value of a given test.

The FDA's Center for Devices and Radiological Health regulates medical devices sold in the United States.[45] There are 2 options the manufacturer of a medical device may take when applying for approval to market by the FDA. The Premarket Approval application option requires a manufacturer to submit valid clinical data to support claims made for the submitted device.[43] During 2016, the FDA approved 34 original Premarket Approval submissions.[46] The other option is the Premarket Notification 510(k) process (aka 510(k)), which requires no such clinical data to support marketing claims.[43] Here, the manufacturer need only show that the submitted device is at least as safe and effective, that is, substantially equivalent to a device that was legally marketed before May 28, 1976. The legally marketed device to which equivalence is drawn is commonly referred to as the "predicate." Because the evidentiary burden is less stringent for the 510(k) process compared with Premarket Approval, most manufacturers use the 510(k) process to obtain marketing clearance (222 devices cleared during January 2017).[47]

Of the adjunctive methodologies discussed herein, only vital stain-based and light-based adjuncts have been cleared for marketing by the FDA. The predicate for the first light-based adjunct to be used in dentistry was a similar device used to illuminate the cervix,[48] and all subsequent light-based adjuncts (**Table 4**) have received FDA clearance in a similar manner.[29–35,37,48–56]

FDA regulation of the recently developed molecular-based adjuncts is less clearly defined. Although the FDA acknowledges it has statutory authority to regulate molecular-based adjuncts, it has yet to release formal regulatory guidance.[57] As a consequence, ongoing FDA oversite over these newly released adjunctive tests is sporadic.

Table 2
Available cytology-based, vital stained-based and light-based adjunctive diagnostic technologies

	Product	Contact	Comments
Cytology based	OralCDx Brush Test	CDx Diagnostics, Suffern, NY	CLIA certified
	CytID	Forward Science, Houston, TX	Liquid cytology sampling assessed by contract pathologist
	MOP	PCG Molecular, Cumming, GA	No response to email inquiry by author
Vital staining based	Toluidine chloride stain (component of ViziLite Plus with TBlue)	Den-Mat Holdings, LLC, Lompoc, CA	Considered a device by the FDA
	OraBlu	AdDent, Inc, Danbury, CT	Considered a device by the FDA
Light-based	ViziLite TBlue	Den-Mat Holdings, LLC, Lompoc, CA	Chemiluminescent generated light source (average wavelength 490–510 nm)
	Microlux DL	AdDent, Inc, Danbury, CT	Battery-powered light source similar to ViziLite light component
	VELscope Vx	LED Dental, White Rock, British Columbia, Canada	LED generated light source (400–460 nm), combined with optical filtration of the viewfinder to enhance natural tissue fluorescence
	Sapphire Plus	Den-Mat Holdings, LLC, Lompoc, CA	Similar to VELscope Vx
	Identafi	DentalEZ, Malvern, PA	White light used for COE Amber light used to highlight superficial vascular architecture Violet light used in conjunction with Identifi Eyewear to assess tissue fluorescence
	Bio/Screen	AdDent, Inc, Danbury, CT	Similar to VELscope Vx
	DOE SE Kit	DentLight Inc, Plano, TX	White light used for COE Violet light used in conjunction with fluorescent loupe filters to assess tissue fluorescence
	OralID	Forward Science, Houston, TX	Eyewear to assess tissue fluorescence.
	ViziLite PRO	Den-Mat Holdings, LLC, Lompoc, CA	Similar to VELscope Vx

Abbreviations: CLIA, clinical laboratory improvement amendments; COE, conventional oral examination; FDA, US Food and Drug Administration; LED, light-emitting diode.
   Data from Refs.[29–37]

Table 3
Available molecular-based adjuncts to diagnose OPMLs/OPC

Product	Company	Biomarkers Assessed
OraRisk HPV Complete Genotype and the	OralDNALabs Eden Prairie, MN	HPV strains: 2a, 6, 11, 16, 18, 26, 30, 31, 32, 33, 34, 35, 39, 40, 41, 42, 43, 44, 45, 49, 51, 52, 53, 54, 55, 56, 57, 58, 59, 60, 61, 62, 64, 66, 67, 68, 69, 70, 71, 72, 73, 74, 75, 76, 77, 80, 81, 82, 83, 84, 89
OraRisk HPV 16/18/HR	OralDNALabs Eden Prairie, MN	HPV strains: 16, 18, 31, 33, 35, 39, 45, 51, 52, 56, 58, 59, 66, 68
MOP	PCG Molecular Cumming, GA	HPV, cellular changes No response to email inquiry by author
SaliMark OSCC	PeriRx, LLC Broomall, PA	DUSP1, SAT, and OAZ1

Abbreviations: HPV, human papilloma virus; OPC, oral and oropharyngeal cancer; OPML, oral pre-malignant lesions.
   Data from Refs.[39–42]

Cytology-Based Adjuncts

Available since 1999, the Oral CDx BrushTest is specifically marketed to the dental professional to "test common oral spots (subtle red or white spots) that may appear in your mouth from time to time."[58] As such, it is a case assessment adjunct. This adjunctive test is a refinement of the Pap smear technique used in gynecology, in which a special sampling brush is used to harvest a full transepithelial specimen that is forwarded to a centralized laboratory for assessment. The appropriate CDT code to use is D7288, "brush biopsy – transepithelial sample collection."[22] At the laboratory, a sophisticated computer protocol is used to assist the pathologist to render a final report. Variants of this technology (WATS[3D], EndoCDx TNE—Transnasal Esophagoscopy, EndoCDx LP—Laryngeal) are marketed to gastroenterologists and otolaryngologists.[59]

Tested lesions that receive a "positive" or "atypical" result with the BrushTest should undergo a scalpel biopsy to determine the definitive diagnosis. Proponents of this adjunctive technique note its favorable positive predictive value and negative predictive value, and feel it allows the practitioner to easily and reliably assess innocuous lesions for benignity, precancer, and cancer, especially for patients hesitant to

Box 1
Parameters of an ideal diagnostic adjunct

1. Simple, inexpensive, safe, and acceptable to the public

2. Detect early disease

3. Detect lesions likely to progress

4. Detect lesions which are manageable

5. Have a high positive predictive value and a low false-negative value

Adapted from Lingen MW, Kalmar JR, Karrison T, et al. Critical evaluation of diagnostic aids for the detection of oral cancer. Oral Oncol 2008;44:10–22; with permission.

Table 4
US Food and Drug Administration premarket notification 510(k) pedigree for available light-based adjuncts

Product	Applicable 510(k)	Date
Speculite (predicate gynecologic illumination device)	K853257	12/27/1985
	K963391	12/12/1997
ViziLite Plus with TBlue	K003995	3/16/2001
	K012070	11/27/2001
	K033033	1/31/2005
	K080043	4/04/2008
Microlux DL	K041614	4/04/2005
	K072309	11/19/2007
VELscope Vx	K060920	4/27/2006
	K070523	4/05/2007
	K102083	11/18/2010
Sapphire Plus	K073483	4/03/2008
Identafi	K082603	12/12/2008
	K090135	2/17/2009
BioScreen	K082668	1/23/2009
DOE SE Kit	K101140	7/15/2010
OralID	K123169	1/13/2013
ViziLite PRO	K082668	1/23/2009

Data from Refs.[29–35,37,48–56]

undergo biopsy.[11,60–63] It may also be useful to initially assess a patient with multiple lesions throughout the mouth, where the attainment of multiple biopsies may be impractical.[25]

Others contend the BrushTest represents an unnecessary intermediate step, because all "positive" or "atypical" results must be biopsied to determine the actual diagnosis.[25,64,65] Furthermore, most sensitivity and specificity values for the BrushTest were calculated predominantly by comparing the efficacy of the test in assessing clinically suspicious, not innocuous, lesions to traditional biopsy.[25,66] Furthermore, a "negative" BrushTest result, although reassuring, is not diagnostic for a persistent lesion.[67,68] The CytID case assessment adjunct uses a liquid cytology sampling technique whereby the harvested cells are placed in a liquid medium for transport to the laboratory. The recommendation for use is similar to that of the previously described Oral CDx BrushTest, for assessing lesions when biopsy is not warranted or possible.[38] The appropriate CDT code to use is D7287, "oral cytologybrush."[22] The use of liquid cytology is claimed to provide a more accurate sampling compared with the Oral CDx BrushTest.[69,70] Tested lesions that receive a "malignancy" or "atypical" result with CytID must undergo a scalpel biopsy to determine the definitive diagnosis.[71]

Vital Stain-Based Adjuncts

Vital staining with toluidine blue (TB) has been advocated as a method to assess suspicious mucosal lesions for decades.[60,72,73] It is metachromatic dye of the thiazine group that has an affinity to bind with DNA. Applied topically, TB selectively stains rapidly dividing tissues such as neoplastic, inflammatory, and regenerative epithelial tissues and exposed connective tissue.[11,60,67] Its use has been advocated by some as a technique to monitor OPMLs for progression, assess suspect lesion margins, and accomplish follow-up on patients who have undergone cancer treatment.[25,74,75] False-positive results are common and primarily associated with inflammatory lesions and healing ulcers, which also have a high cellular metabolic rate.[25,60,76]

TB is currently not cleared by the FDA as a stand-alone adjunctive screening aid. It is cleared for marketing as a case assessment marking aid to the ViziLite TBlue (Den-Mat Holdings, LLC, Lompoc, CA), Bio/Screen (AdDent, Inc, Danbury, CT), and Micro-Lux DL (AdDent, Inc) adjunctive aids, where it may be used to further enhance the marking of an area initially identified via the companion light-based adjunct.[29,36] The appropriate CDT code to apply when using TB is D0431, "adjunctive pre-diagnostic test that aids in detection of mucosal abnormalities including premalignant and malignant lesions, not to include cytology or biopsy procedures."[22]

Light-Based Adjuncts

The development of the light-based adjuncts represents the culmination of years of medical research investigating the unique absorbance and reflectance characteristics of dysplastic or malignant mucosal tissues.[77–85] Advocates contend these devices are easy to use and enhance the clinician's ability to discover OPML and OPC by improving lesion visualization and potentially revealing lesions missed by the COE.[86,87] Unfortunately, the majority of studies addressing their efficacy have been limited to case reports and proof-of-concept trials, often by experienced examiners who have a higher degree of confidence in distinguishing between suspicious and nonsuspicious lesions.[25,88] The light-based adjuncts can be categorized into 2 basic groups according to the manner in which a specific spectra of light is used to interrogate the reflective properties of the tissue.

The ViziLite TBlue and Microlux DL use a blue-white light (spectral wavelength of 430 and 580 nm) to interrogate the tissues. For the ViziLite TBlue product, the blue-white light is generated through reaction between acetylsalicylic acid and hydrogen peroxide (chemiluminescence), whereas the blue-white light for the Microlux DL product is produced by a battery-powered light-emitting diode.[25] The protocol for both regimens entails the use of a 60-second prerinse with a 1% acetic acid solution to remove the surface glycoprotein layer and cause cellular dehydration, to improve the exposure of cellular elements to the blue-white light.[25,88] The examination takes place in a darkened room or with the use of special eyewear. The premise is that normal cells absorb the blue-white light whereas dysplastic cells with abnormal nuclei and high nuclear/cytoplasmic ratios reflect the blue-white back to the examiner as "aceto-white."[67,88,89]

The VELscope Vx (LED Dental, White Rock, British Columbia, Canada), Sapphire Plus (Den-Mat Holdings, LLC), Identafi (DentalEZ, Malvern, PA), BioScreen (AdDent, Inc), DOE Oral Exam System (DentLight, Inc, Plano, TX), OralID (Forward Science, Houston, TX), and ViziLite PRO (Den-Mat Holdings, LLC) use light spectra in the 390 to 460 nm range to interrogate the tissue autofluorescent character of the mucosal tissues.[25] All of these devices use a narrow band filter (either in the device viewfinder or via eyewear) to emphasize the autofluorescent character of the lesion. The principle concept is that the natural autofluorescent character of dysplastic or malignant tissues is different from normal tissues. Dysplastic or carcinogenic tissues are associated with increased collagen destruction, nuclear/cytoplasmic ratio, and angiogenesis.[67,86,90] The net result of these phenomena is a decrease in natural fluorophore concentration and an increased absorption and scattering of light.[88] Normal or healthy tissue appears pale green using autofluorescence, whereas suspect tissues appear dark (loss of fluorescence).[91] The Identafi adds an additional green-amber light (545 nm) to better visualize the increase in angiogenesis associated with carcinoma.[92,93]

Although the design parameters (eg, light source, light filtration, disposability) and visualization characteristics vary among the light-based adjuncts, the principle underlying their use is similar and they are all cleared for marketing by the FDA as illumination devices.[94] All are marketed to assist the practitioner in discovering new or potentially overlooked mucosal abnormalities. Some are also marketed to assist the surgeon in defining appropriate surgical margins for excision.[60,95]

Although light-based adjuncts do offer the clinician a different perspective to view a lesion (eg, assessment utility), their value and efficacy as screening adjuncts remains unproven.[88,91,96,97] Rashid and Warnakulasuriya[88] reviewed 14 published reports addressing the effectiveness of the VELscope, ViziLite, and Microlux DL adjuncts (**Table 5**) and concluded they demonstrate poor specificity and lack the ability to discriminate between high-risk and low-risk lesions. They further noted that the Vizi-Lite and MicroLux DL preferentially highlighted keratotic lesions over red lesions and the VELscope revealed a lack of fluorescence in benign keratosis and inflammatory lesions. They concluded there is insufficient evidence to validate their efficacy as screening adjuncts.

OHPs choosing to use any of the available visualization adjuncts in assessing their patients should understand their limitations and ensure an appropriate referral and/or biopsy is accomplished for any lesion deemed suspicious. The appropriate CDT code to apply when using one of these adjunctive aids is D0431, "adjunctive pre-diagnostic test that aids in detection of mucosal abnormalities including premalignant and malignant lesions, not to include cytology or biopsy procedures."[22]

Molecular-Based Adjuncts
***

Saliva has become an increasingly popular medium to assess for potential biomarkers associated with OPML and OPC.[98–100] Potential biomarkers associated with OPC include nonorganic compounds; proteins and peptides; DNA, messenger RNA, microRNA; carbohydrates; and other metabolites.[98] The number of potentially useful biomarkers has increased significantly over the past decade. Sivadasan and colleagues[101] recently reported the human salivary proteome contains more than 3400 proteins, of which 808 have been differentially expressed in OPC.

Advancements in our ability to map the molecular mechanisms underlying the pathogenesis of OPC should lead to the development of improved diagnostic and therapeutic interventions targeting OPC.[25,100] The goal of developing a reliable salivary test or tests to assess for OPML and OPC remains a significant challenge and is complicated by our inability to effectively compare the numerous published studies, owing to variabilities in study design and interpretation (eg, sampling techniques, processing techniques, cutoff points, etc).[98,100,102,103] Another underappreciated

Table 5					
Efficacy of 3 light-based screening adjuncts					
Adjunct	**# Articles**	**Sensitivity (%)**	**Specificity (%)**	**Positive Predictive Value (%)**	**Negative Predictive Value (%)**
ViziLite Plus	12	0–100	0–78	18–100	0–100
Microlux DL	1	78	71	37	94
VELscope	12	30–100	15–100	6–59	57–100

Adapted from Rashid A, Warnakulasuriya S. The use of light-based (optical) detection systems as adjuncts in the detection of oral cancer and oral potentially malignant disorders: a systematic review. J Oral Pathol Med 2015;44:307–28; with permission.

confounder is the molecular heterogeneity of OPC itself.[104–106] Despite these hurdles, various molecular-based adjunctive tests (see **Table 3**) have been introduced to the dental marketplace as putative aids to assess for OPC or the risk of developing OPC and are discussed briefly.

The OraRisk HPV Complete Genotype and the OraRisk HPV 16/18/HR (OralDNA-Labs Eden Prairie, MN) are 2 polymerase chain reaction–based tests available for determining the presence of human papilloma virus (HPV).[39,40] The OraRisk HPV Complete Genotype utility screens for 51 strains of HPV, whereas the OraRisk HPV 16/18/HR utility tests for 20 oncogenic HPVs, to include HPV 16 and HPV 18.

The prognostic value of current or persistent HPV detection in oral rinses to predict the risk for oral squamous cell carcinoma is unknown.[107–110] The cost–benefit value of this test is debatable, because an estimated 10,500 individual would need to be tested to detect 1 case of OPC.[109] More problematic is the fact that high-risk HPV prevalence is estimated to be 4.0% among adults aged 18 to 69 (men, 6.8%; women, 1.2%) and, to date, there are no available interventions to reduce or prevent the downstream future development of HPV associated OPC.[109] Ultimately, the benefit to risk of using this test as a screening utility may not be favorable, because it is not predictive of progression to OPC and may produce significant anxiety for those who screen positive for a high-risk HPV.[110]

The MOP screening test from PCG Molecular claims to test for oral cancer risk earlier than traditional testing methods by assessing the presence of 3 parameters: HPV infection, cellular abnormalities, and DNA damage.[111] The test essentially combines cytology, HPV testing, and an unspecified form of DNA assessment. It consists of a 30-second gargle and rinse to obtain the sample, which is sent to the company for assessment. Patients who test positive "will need to be evaluated by an ENT or an oral surgeon depending on the levels found." The website also alludes to litigious risk if one does not use the product, based on the following comment, "By offering the MOP test both the responsibility and the liability for early detection is placed on the patient. If patients decline the test, practitioners have their written directive on file. With cases expected to increase dramatically over the next 20 years, practitioners are well advised to have such safeguards in place."[112]

Information on this test seems to be restricted to its promotional website and there seems to be no published literature addressing the value or validity of this testing protocol as a screening utility. In contrast, the National Cancer Institute notes there are no currently recommended screening methods similar to a Pap test for detecting cell changes in the oropharyngeal tissues caused by HPV infection.[113]

The SaliMark OSCC adjunctive test (PeriRx, LLC, Broomall, PA) is a recently introduced case assessment product intended to help the practitioner stratify the risk of malignancy for a clinically discovered oral lesion.[42] The premise is that, by determining the levels of messenger RNAs for the genes DUSP1, SAT, and OAZ1, along with the messenger RNAs for the housekeeping genes MTATP6 and RPL30, oral lesions at high risk for being OPC may be discriminated from low-risk oral lesions.[114] In a study of 168 patients with oral lesions suspicious for cancer, out of which 24 had cancer, the sensitivity and specificity of the SaliMark OSCC adjunctive test was determined to be 91.7% and 59.0%, respectively.[114] The results of the study essentially establish proof of concept, but have not been validated independently. More important, the performance of this product to assess the variety of nonmalignant oral lesions encountered in general practice is unknown.

The SaliMark OSCC adjunctive test is marketed as a negative predictor, whereby patients with moderate or high test results should be referred for further evaluation and/or biopsy, whereas patients with low-risk results should be followed up to ensure resolution. This protocol for lesion assessment has been proposed by some as a method to reduce unnecessary referrals and biopsies.[115] Such an approach seems to assume that the only purpose of a biopsy or referral is to determine the presence of malignancy and conflicts with the foundational principle that a referral and/or biopsy is indicated for any lesion for which the practitioner cannot confidently establish the diagnosis.

SUMMARY

The most important prognostic factor in predicting the outcome of OPC continues to be the stage at which it is diagnosed. Approximately 70% of patients with OPC are diagnosed with late stage disease and patient-related delay is a major factor in late stage diagnosis. Efforts to increase the patient's ability and desire to obtain an oral examination on a regular basis should be undertaken.

The OHP often has the opportunity to identify OPC at its earliest stage. When patients present for care, OHPs should accomplish a disciplined and thorough COE to discover any abnormalities, not just OPC. Any suspicious or equivocal lesion should be referred for further assessment or undergo biopsy, whereas innocuous lesions should be reevaluated within 4 weeks and referred for further assessment or undergo biopsy if still present.

The evidence for use of adjunctive devices to screen for and/or identify OPCs and OPMLs at their earliest stage remains low. Clinicians are cautioned to consider the available scientific literature, objective measures of performance, and available evidence-based guidelines in determining the value of using such devices in clinical practice.

REFERENCES

1. Siegel RL, Miller KD, Jemal A. Cancer Statistics, 2017. CA Cancer J Clin 2016; 67:7–30.
2. Li L, Morse DE, Katz RV. What constitutes a proper routine oral cancer examination for patients at low risk? Findings from a Delphi survey. Oral Surg Oral Med Oral Pathol Oral Radiol 2013;116:e379–86.
3. Seoane J, Alvarez-Novoa P, Gomez I, et al. Early oral cancer diagnosis: the Aarhus statement perspective. A systematic review and meta-analysis. Head Neck 2016;38(Suppl 1):E2182–9.
4. Silverman S Jr, Kerr AR, Epstein JB. Oral and pharyngeal cancer control and early detection. J Cancer Educ 2010;25:279–81.
5. Stefanuto P, Doucet JC, Robertson C. Delays in treatment of oral cancer: a review of the current literature. Oral Surg Oral Med Oral Pathol Oral Radiol 2014;117:424–9.
6. Varela-Centelles P, López-Cedrún JL, Fernández-Sanromán J, et al. Key points and time intervals for early diagnosis in symptomatic oral cancer: a systematic review. Int J Oral Maxillofac Surg 2017;46:1–10.
7. Jensen AR, Nellemann HM, Overgaard J. Tumor progression in waiting time for radiotherapy in head and neck cancer. Radiother Oncol 2007;84:5–10.
8. Waaijer A, Terhaard CHJ, Dehnad H, et al. Waiting times for radiotherapy: consequences of volume increase for the TCP in oropharyngeal carcinoma. Radiother Oncol 2003;66:271–6.
9. Holmes JD, Dierks EJ, Homer LD, et al. Is detection of oral and oropharyngeal squamous cancer by a dental health care provider associated with a lower stage at diagnosis? J Oral Maxillofac Surg 2003;61:285–91.

10. National Cancer Institute. SEER Cancer Statistics Review 1973-1993. Available at: https://seer.cancer.gov/archive/csr/1973_1993/oralcav.pdf. Accessed May 5, 2017.

11. Güneri P, Epstein JB. Late stage diagnosis of oral cancer: components and possible solutions. Oral Oncol 2014;50:1131–6.

12. Friedrich RE. Delay in diagnosis and referral patterns of 646 patients with oral and maxillofacial cancer: a report from a single institution in Hamburg, Germany. Anticancer Res 2010;30:1833–6.

13. Peacock ZS, Pogrel MA, Schmidt BL. Exploring the reasons for delay in treatment of oral cancer. J Am Dent Assoc 2008;139:1346–52.

14. Goy J, Hall SF, Feldman-Stewart D, et al. Diagnostic delay and disease stage in head and neck cancer: a systematic review. Laryngoscope 2009;119:889–98.

15. Scott SE, Grunfeld EA, McGurk M. Patient's delay in oral cancer: a systematic review. Community Dent Oral Epidemiol 2006;34:337–43.

16. Noonan B. Understanding the reasons why patients delay seeking treatment for oral cancer symptoms from a primary health care professional: an integrative literature review. Eur J Oncol Nurs 2014;18:118–24.

17. Gallup. One-third of Americans Haven't Visited dentist in past year. Available at: http://www.gallup.com/poll/168716/one-third-americans-haven-visited-dentist-past-year.aspx. Accessed May 5, 2017.

18. Netuveli G, Sheiham A, Watt RG. Does the 'inverse screening law' apply to oral cancer screening and regular dental check-ups? J Med Screen 2006;13:47–50.

19. Ford PJ, Farah CS. Early detection and diagnosis of oral cancer: strategies for improvement. J Cancer Policy 2013;1:e2–7.

20. Brouha XD, Tromp DM, Koole R, et al. Professional delay in head and neck cancer patients: analysis of the diagnostic pathway. Oral Oncol 2007;43:551–6.

21. Lydiatt DD. Cancer of the oral cavity and medical malpractice. Laryngoscope 2002;112:816–9.

22. American Dental Association. CDT 2017 dental procedure codes. Chicago: American Dental Association; 2016.

23. Mathew B, Sankaranarayanan R, Sunilkumar KB, et al. Reproducibility and validity of oral visual inspection by trained health workers in the detection of oral precancer and cancer. Br J Cancer 1997;76:390–4.

24. Fischer DJ, Epstein JB, Morton TH, et al. Interobserver reliability in the histopathologic diagnosis of oral pre-malignant and malignant lesions. J Oral Pathol Med 2004;33:65–70.

25. Lingen MW, Kalmar JR, Karrison T, et al. Critical evaluation of diagnostic aids for the detection of oral cancer. Oral Oncol 2008;44:10–22.

26. Mignogna MD, Fedele S, Lo Russo L, et al. Oral and pharyngeal cancer: lack of prevention and early detection by health care providers. Eur J Cancer Prev 2001;10:381–3.

27. National Cancer Institute. Oral cancer screening (PDQ®), description of the evidence significance. Available at: http://www.cancer.gov/cancertopics/pdq/screening/oral/HealthProfessional/page2. Accessed May 15, 2017.

28. CDx Diagnositics. OralCDx. Available at: http://cdxdiagnostics.com/OralCDx.html. Accessed May 15, 2017.

29. US Food and Drug Administration (FDA) website. Premarket notification K033033. Available at: http://www.accessdata.fda.gov/cdrh_docs/pdf3/K033033.pdf. Accessed May 15, 2017.

30. US Food and Drug Administration (FDA) website. Premarket notification K041614. Available at: http://www.accessdata.fda.gov/cdrh_docs/pdf4/K041614.pdf. Accessed May 15, 2017.
31. US Food and Drug Administration (FDA) website. Premarket notification K073483. Available at: https://www.accessdata.fda.gov/cdrh_docs/pdf7/K073483.pdf. Accessed May 15, 2017.
32. US Food and Drug Administration (FDA) website. Premarket notification K082668. Available at: https://www.accessdata.fda.gov/cdrh_docs/pdf8/K082668.pdf. Accessed May 15, 2017.
33. US Food and Drug Administration (FDA) website. Premarket notification K090135. Available at: https://www.accessdata.fda.gov/cdrh_docs/pdf9/K090135.pdf. Accessed May 15, 2017.
34. US Food and Drug Administration (FDA) website. Premarket notification K101140. Available at: https://www.accessdata.fda.gov/cdrh_docs/pdf10/K101140.pdf. Accessed May 15, 2017.
35. US Food and Drug Administration (FDA) website. Premarket notification K102083. Available at: https://www.accessdata.fda.gov/cdrh_docs/pdf10/K102083.pdf. Accessed May 15, 2017.
36. US Food and Drug Administration (FDA) website. Premarket notification K121282. Available at: https://www.accessdata.fda.gov/cdrh_docs/pdf12/K121282.pdf. Accessed May 15, 2017.
37. US Food and Drug Administration (FDA) website. Premarket notification K123169. Available at: https://www.accessdata.fda.gov/cdrh_docs/pdf12/K123169.pdf. Accessed May 15, 2017.
38. Forward Science. CytID. Available at: http://www.forwardscience.com/cytid. Accessed May 15, 2017.
39. OralDNA Labs. OraRisk® HPV 16/18/HR testing from OralDNA Labs. Available at: https://www.oraldna.com/hpv-testing.html. Accessed May 15, 2017.
40. OralDNA Labs. OraRisk® HPV, Complete Genotyping Testing From OralDNA Labs. Available at: https://www.oraldna.com/oral-hpv-testing.html. Accessed May 15, 2017.
41. Pcgmolecular. What does MOP™ screen for? Available at: http://pcgmolecular.com/mop-test/. Accessed May 15, 2017.
42. PeriRx. SaliMark OSCC. Available at: http://perirx.com/products/. Accessed May 15, 2017.
43. Huber MA. Adjunctive diagnostic aids in oral cancer screening: an update. Tex Dent J 2012;129:471–80.
44. US Food and Drug Administration (FDA) website. Clinical laboratory improvement amendments (CLIA). Available at: https://www.fda.gov/MedicalDevices/DeviceRegulationandGuidance/IVDRegulatoryAssistance/ucm124105.htm. Accessed May 15, 2017.
45. US Food and Drug Administration (FDA) website. Statement of FDA Mission. Available at: https://www.fda.gov/downloads/AboutFDA/ReportsManualsForms/Reports/BudgetReports/UCM298331.pdf. Accessed May 15, 2017.
46. US Food and Drug Administration (FDA) website. Devices Approved in 2016. Available at: https://www.fda.gov/MedicalDevices/ProductsandMedicalProcedures/DeviceApprovalsandClearances/PMAApprovals/ucm484383.htm. Accessed May 15, 2017.
47. US Food and Drug Administration (FDA) website. 510(k) Premarket Notification. Available at: https://www.accessdata.fda.gov/scripts/cdrh/cfdocs/cfPMN/pmn.cfm. Accessed May 15, 2017.

48. US Food and Drug Administration (FDA) website. Premarket notification K853257. Available at: https://www.accessdata.fda.gov/scripts/cdrh/cfdocs/cfPMN/pmn. cfm?ID=K853257. Accessed May 15, 2017.

49. US Food and Drug Administration (FDA) website. Premarket notification K963391. Available at: https://www.accessdata.fda.gov/scripts/cdrh/cfdocs/cfPMN/pmn. cfm?ID=K963391. Accessed May 15, 2017.

50. US Food and Drug Administration (FDA) website. Premarket notification K003995. Available at: https://www.accessdata.fda.gov/scripts/cdrh/cfdocs/cfPMN/pmn. cfm?ID=K003995. Accessed May 15, 2017.

51. US Food and Drug Administration (FDA) website. Premarket notification K012070. Available at: https://www.accessdata.fda.gov/scripts/cdrh/cfdocs/cfPMN/pmn. cfm?ID=K012070. Accessed May 15, 2017.

52. US Food and Drug Administration (FDA) website. Premarket notification K080043. Available at: https://www.accessdata.fda.gov/scripts/cdrh/cfdocs/cfPMN/pmn. cfm?ID=K080043. Accessed May 15, 2017.

53. US Food and Drug Administration (FDA) website. Premarket notification K072309. Available at: https://www.accessdata.fda.gov/scripts/cdrh/cfdocs/cfPMN/pmn. cfm?ID=K072309. Accessed May 15, 2017.

54. US Food and Drug Administration (FDA) website. Premarket notification K060920. Available at: https://www.accessdata.fda.gov/scripts/cdrh/cfdocs/cfPMN/pmn. cfm?ID=K060920. Accessed May 15, 2017.

55. US Food and Drug Administration (FDA) website. Premarket notification K070523. Available at: https://www.accessdata.fda.gov/scripts/cdrh/cfdocs/cfPMN/pmn. cfm?ID=K070523. Accessed May 15, 2017.

56. US Food and Drug Administration (FDA) website. Premarket notification K082603. Available at: https://www.accessdata.fda.gov/scripts/cdrh/cfdocs/cfPMN/pmn. cfm?ID=K082603. Accessed May 15, 2017.

57. US Food and Drug Administration (FDA) website. Discussion paper on laboratory developed tests (LDTs) January 13, 2017. Available at: https://www.fda.gov/ downloads/MedicalDevices/ProductsandMedicalProcedures/InVitroDiagnostics/ LaboratoryDevelopedTests/UCM536965.pdf. Accessed May 15, 2017.

58. OralCDx. What is the OralCDx Brush Test? Available at: https://thebrushtest. com/what-is-the-brushtest/. Accessed May 15, 2017.

59. CDx Diagnostics. CDx Technology. Available at: http://cdxdiagnostics.com/ CDx_technology.html. Accessed May 15, 2017.

60. Chhabra N, Chhabra S, Sapra N. Diagnostic modalities for squamous cell carcinoma: an extensive review of literature-considering toluidine blue as a useful adjunct. J Maxillofac Oral Surg 2015;14:188–200.

61. Eisen D, Frist S. The relevance of the high positive predictive value of the oral brush biopsy. Oral Oncol 2005;41:753–5.

62. Mehrotra R, Mishra S, Singh M, et al. The efficacy of oral brush biopsy with computer-assisted analysis in identifying precancerous and cancerous lesions. Head Neck Oncol 2011;24(3):39.

63. Scheifele C, Schmidt-Westhausen AM, Dietrich T, et al. The sensitivity and specificity of the oral CDx technique: evaluation of 103 cases. Oral Oncol 2004;40: 824–8.

64. Bhoopathi V, Kabani S, Mascarenhas AK. Low positive predictive value of the oral brush biopsy in detecting dysplastic oral lesions. Cancer 2009;115: 1036–40.

65. Fedele S. Diagnostic aids in the screening of oral cancer. Head Neck Oncol 2009;1:5.

66. Slater LJ. Oral brush biopsy: false positives redux. Oral Surg Oral Med Oral Pathol Oral Radiol Endod 2004;97:419.
67. Cheng YS, Rees T, Wright J. Updates regarding diagnostic adjuncts for oral squamous cell carcinoma. Tex Dent J 2015;132:538–49.
68. Koch FP, Kunkel M, Biesterfeld S, et al. Diagnostic efficiency of differentiating small cancerous and precancerous lesions using mucosal brush smears of the oral cavity–a prospective and blinded study. Clin Oral Investig 2011;15: 763–9.
69. Hayama FH, Motta AC, Silva Ade P, et al. Liquid-based preparations versus conventional cytology: specimen adequacy and diagnostic agreement in oral lesions. Med Oral Patol Oral Cir Bucal 2005;10:115–22.
70. Navone R, Burlo P, Pich A, et al. The impact of liquid-based oral cytology on the diagnosis of oral squamous dysplasia and carcinoma. Cytopathology 2007;18: 356–60.
71. Forward Science. CytID, Technology. Available at: http://www.forwardscience. com/cytid/technology. Accessed May 15, 2017.
72. Mashberg A. Final evaluation of tolonium chloride rinse for screening of high-risk patients with asymptomatic squamous carcinoma. J Am Dent Assoc 1983;106: 319–23.
73. Silverman S Jr, Migliorati C, Barbosa J. Toluidine blue staining in the detection of oral precancerous and malignant lesions. Oral Surg Oral Med Oral Pathol 1984; 57:379–82.
74. Epstein JB, Güneri P. The adjunctive role of toluidine blue in detection of oral premalignant and malignant lesions. Curr Opin Otolaryngol Head Neck Surg 2009;17:79–87.
75. Zhang L, Williams M, Poh CF, et al. Toluidine blue staining identifies high-risk primary oral premalignant lesions with poor outcome. Cancer Res 2005;65: 8017–21.
76. Richards D. Does toluidine blue detect more oral cancer? Evid Based Dent 2010;11:104–5.
77. De Veld DC, Skurichina M, Witjes MJ, et al. Autofluorescence and diffuse reflectance spectroscopy for oral oncology. Lasers Surg Med 2005;36:356–64.
78. De Veld DC, Witjes MJ, Sterenborg HJ, et al. The status of in vivo autofluorescence spectroscopy and imaging for oral oncology. Oral Oncol 2005;41:117–31.
79. Ebihara A, Krasieva TB, Liaw LH, et al. Detection and diagnosis of oral cancer by light-induced fluorescence. Lasers Surg Med 2003;32:17–24.
80. Koch FP, Kaemmerer PW, Biesterfeld S, et al. Effectiveness of autofluorescence to identify suspicious oral lesions – a prospective, blinded clinical trial. Clin Oral Investig 2011;15:975–82.
81. Onizawa K, Okamura N, Saginoya H, et al. Characterization of autofluorescence in oral squamous cell carcinoma. Oral Oncol 2003;39(2):150–6.
82. Rahman MS, Ingole N, Roblyer D, et al. Evaluation of low-cost, portable imaging system for early detection of oral cancer. Head Neck Oncol 2010;2:10.
83. Roblyer D, Kurachi C, Stepanek V, et al. Objective detection and delineation of oral neoplasia using autofluorescence imaging. Cancer Prev Res 2009;2: 423–31.
84. Svistun E, Alizadeh-Naderi R, El-Naggar A, et al. Vision enhancement system for detection of oral cavity neoplasia based on autofluorescence. Head Neck 2004; 26:205–15.

85. Wang CY, Chiang HK, Chen CT, et al. Diagnosis of oral cancer by light-induced autofluorescence spectroscopy using double excitation wavelengths. Oral Oncol 1999;35:144–50.

86. Lane P, Lam S, Follen M, et al. Oral fluorescence imaging using 405-nm excitation, aiding the discrimination of cancers and precancers by identifying changes in collagen and elastic breakdown and neovascularization in the underlying stroma. Gend Med 2012;9(1 Suppl):78–82.e1-8.

87. Truelove EL, Dean D, Maltby S, et al. Narrow band (light) imaging of oral mucosa in routine dental patients. Part 1: assessment of value in detection of mucosal changes. Gen Dent 2011;59:281–9 [quiz: 290–1, 319–20].

88. Rashid A, Warnakulasuriya S. The use of light-based (optical) detection systems as adjuncts in the detection of oral cancer and oral potentially malignant disorders: a systematic review. J Oral Pathol Med 2015;44:307–28.

89. Huber MA, Bsoul SA, Terezhalmy GT. Acetic acid wash and chemiluminescent illumination as an adjunct to conventional oral soft tissue examination for the detection of dysplasia: a pilot study. Quintessence Int 2004;35:378–84.

90. Sokolov K, Follen M, Richards-Kortum R. Optical spectroscopy for detection of neoplasia. Curr Opin Chem Biol 2002;6:651–8.

91. McNamara KK, Martin BD, Evans EW, et al. The role of direct visual fluorescent examination (VELscope) in routine screening for potentially malignant oral mucosal lesions. Oral Surg Oral Med Oral Pathol Oral Radiol 2012;114:636–43.

92. Lane P, Follen M, MacAulay C. Has fluorescence spectroscopy come of age? A case series of oral precancers and cancers using white light, fluorescent light at 405 nm, and reflected light at 545 nm using the Trimira Identafi 3000. Gend Med 2012;9(1 Suppl):S25–35.

93. Messadi DV, Younai FS, Liu HH, et al. The clinical effectiveness of reflectance optical spectroscopy for the in vivo diagnosis of oral lesions. Int J Oral Sci 2014;6:162–7.

94. Huber MA, Epstein JB. Marketing versus science: a call for evidence-based advertising in dentistry. Oral Surg Oral Med Oral Pathol Oral Radiol 2015;120:541–3.

95. Poh CF, Zhang L, Anderson DW, et al. Fluorescence visualization detection of field alterations in tumor margins of oral cancer patients. Clin Cancer Res 2006;12:6716–22.

96. Patton LL, Epstein JB, Kerr AR. Adjunctive techniques for oral cancer examination and lesion diagnosis: a systematic review of the literature. J Am Dent Assoc 2008;139:896–905.

97. Rethman MP, Carpenter W, Cohen EE, et al. American Dental Association Council on Scientific Affairs Expert Panel on screening for oral squamous cell carcinomas. Evidence-based clinical recommendations regarding screening for oral squamous cell carcinomas. J Am Dent Assoc 2010;141:509–20.

98. Cheng YS, Rees T, Wright J. A review of research on salivary biomarkers for oral cancer detection. Clin Transl Med 2014;3:3.

99. Liu J, Duan Y. Saliva: a potential media for disease diagnostics and monitoring. Oral Oncol 2012;48:569–77.

100. Malik UU, Zarina S, Pennington SR. Oral squamous cell carcinoma: key clinical questions, biomarker discovery, and the role of proteomics. Arch Oral Biol 2016;63:53–65.

101. Sivadasan P, Gupta MK, Sathe GJ, et al. Human salivary proteome–a resource of potential biomarkers for oral cancer. J Proteomics 2015;127(Pt A):89–95.

102. Lingen MW, Pinto A, Mendes RA, et al. Genetics/epigenetics of oral premalignancy: current status and future research. Oral Dis 2011;17(Suppl 1):7–22.
103. Stuani VT, Rubira CM, Sant'Ana AC, et al. Salivary biomarkers as tools for oral squamous cell carcinoma diagnosis: a systematic review. Head Neck 2017; 39:797–811.
104. Almendro V, Marusyk A, Polyak K. Cellular heterogeneity and molecular evolution in cancer. Annu Rev Pathol 2013;8:277–302.
105. Marusyk A, Almendro V, Polyak K. Intra-tumour heterogeneity: a looking glass for cancer? Nat Rev Cancer 2012;12:323–34.
106. McGranahan N, Swanton C. Biological and therapeutic impact of intratumor heterogeneity in cancer evolution. Cancer Cell 2015;27:15–26.
107. Castle PE. Teaching moment: why promising biomarkers do not always translate into clinically useful tests. J Clin Oncol 2014;32:359–61.
108. Chai RC, Lambie D, Verma M, et al. Current trends in the etiology and diagnosis of HPV-related head and neck cancers. Cancer Med 2015;4:596–607.
109. Gillison ML, Chaturvedi AK, Anderson WF, et al. Epidemiology of human papillomavirus-positive head and neck squamous cell carcinoma. J Clin Oncol 2015;33:3235–42.
110. Rettig E, Kiess AP, Fakhry C. The role of sexual behavior in head and neck cancer: implications for prevention and therapy. Expert Rev Anticancer Ther 2015; 15:35–49.
111. PCG Molecular. What does MOP screen for? Available at: http://www.pcgmolecular.com/mop-test/. Accessed May 15, 2017.
112. PCG Molecular. A preventative approach – genetic testing for cancer. Available at: http://pcgmolecular.com/our-approach/. Accessed May 15, 2017.
113. National Cancer Institute. HPV and cancer. Available at: https://www.cancer.gov/about-cancer/causes-prevention/risk/infectious-agents/hpv-fact-sheet. Accessed May 15, 2017.
114. Martin JL, Gottehrer N, Zalesin H, et al. Evaluation of salivary transcriptome markers for the early detection of oral squamous cell cancer in a prospective blinded trial. Compend Contin Educ Dent 2015;36:365–73.
115. Bonne NJ, Wong DT. Salivary biomarker development using genomic, proteomic and metabolomic approaches. Genome Med 2012;4:82.

Surgical Management of Oral Cancer

Rabie M. Shanti, DMD, MD[a,b,*], Bert W. O'Malley Jr, MD[b]

KEYWORDS

- Oral cancer • Mandibulectomy • Maxillectomy • Glossectomy • Neck dissection

KEY POINTS

- Primarily, surgery is the standard of care for early-stage oral cancer.
- Distant metastasis must be ruled out before proceeding with surgical management of an oral cancer.
- Oral cavity squamous cell carcinoma (SCC) is best managed with 1- to 1.5-cm surgical margins.
- There is a survival benefit in performing a selective neck dissection in early-stage oral cavity SCC.

ROLE OF SURGERY IN HEAD AND NECK CANCER MANAGEMENT

Today, most head and neck cancer subsites, such as the larynx, hypopharynx, nasopharynx, and oropharynx, are treated with radiation therapy (XRT) with or without chemotherapy as a primary treatment modality. Recent advances with transoral robotic surgery (TORS) have significantly impacted the management of cancers of the oropharynx. Surgery is reserved for the salvage of recurrent tumors that occur within the head and neck in the absence of distant (ie, lung, liver) metastasis. The results of the Veterans Administration Larynx Trial published in 1991 identified induction chemotherapy followed by XRT provided the same 2-year survival as conventional laryngectomy plus adjuvant XRT.[1] Furthermore, in this study, the larynx was preserved in 64% of patients in the chemoradiotherapy (CRT) arm of the study.[1] Today, roughly 30% to 40% of patients who undergo primary CRT for laryngeal squamous cell carcinoma (SCC) will experience treatment failure with locoregional recurrence of their tumor, and in the absence of distant metastasis, these patients will go on to require either a partial or a total laryngectomy (**Fig. 1**).[2,3]

Disclosure Statement: The authors have no relevant disclosures.
[a] Department of Oral and Maxillofacial Surgery and Pharmacology, University of Pennsylvania School of Dental Medicine, 240 S 40th Street #122, Philadelphia, PA 19104, USA; [b] Department of Otorhinolaryngology/Head and Neck Surgery, Perelman School of Medicine University of Pennsylvania, 3400 Civic Center Boulevard, Philadelphia, PA 19104, USA
* Corresponding author. Department of Otorhinolaryngology/Head and Neck Surgery, University of Pennsylvania Perelman School of Medicine, 3400 Civic Center Boulevard, Philadelphia, PA 19104.
E-mail address: rabie.shanti@uphs.upenn.edu

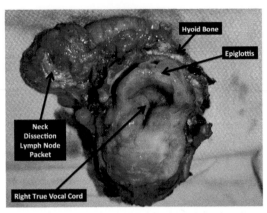

Fig. 1. Total laryngectomy specimen, which includes the epiglottis, vocal cords, thyroid cartilage, cricoid cartilage, hyoid bone, upper tracheal rings, and neck dissection lymph node packet.

Contrary to the larynx, the oropharynx as a subsite has been shown to benefit from primary surgery with adjuvant therapy as needed. However, the extirpation of advanced malignant neoplasms of the oropharynx traditionally required open approaches that required invasive transcervical surgical approaches, such as lip-split with mandibulotomy/mandibulectomy (**Fig. 2**). Although transcervical approaches such as the lip-split mandibulotomy can appear quite graphic and morbid, the benefit from extirpation of SCC of the oropharynx results in the ability to achieve locoregional disease control with a 20% reduction in locoregional recurrence in comparison to primary CRT.[4] This benefit in locoregional disease control and overall survival provided by primary surgery in oropharyngeal SCC served the basis for significant surgical innovation in head and neck surgery. In search of less invasive surgical approaches, Hockstein and colleagues[5] reported on the potential of the da Vinci surgical system (Intuitive Surgical, Inc, Sunnyvale, CA, USA) system in performing extirpative operations that would have classically required a transcervical access–type approach. In 2009, the US Food and Drug Administration approved the da Vinci robotic surgery

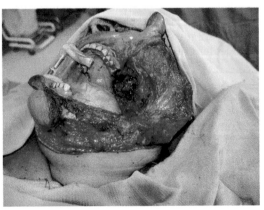

Fig. 2. Intraoperative photograph following tumor extirpation requiring lip-split mandibulectomy.

for surgery of the oropharynx through the work of the senior author (B.W.O.) and Gregory S. Weinstein, MD from the University of Pennsylvania. Today, TORS allows surgeons, through the use of special retractors (**Fig. 3**) and sophisticated technology, the ability to surgically treat tumors within the oropharynx, hypopharynx, and upper portions of the larynx that would have been otherwise treated with primary CRT or substantially more invasive traditional access approaches, such as lip-split mandibulotomy.

Unlike all other head and neck subsites, oral SCC ideally should be managed with primary surgery with the possibility of adjuvant XRT with or without chemotherapy, depending on the presence of certain high-risk pathologic features. The current evidence supports that when safe to do so from a surgical and medical perspective, primary surgery should be attempted whenever possible to provide patients with the greatest chance of cure. This issue of the *Dental Clinics of North America* is devoted to oral cancer; therefore, the remainder of this article focuses on the role of surgery in the management of oral SCC, because this neoplasm constitutes 90% of oral cavity malignancies.

Today, it is unknown why oral SCC is so responsive to primary surgery in comparison to primary XRT or primary CRT, which is not necessarily the case for other subsites, such as the larynx, hypopharynx, or nasopharynx, and in certain cases, oropharyngeal SCC. However, even though surgery is the ideal primary treatment modality for oral SCC, one must not underestimate the limitations of surgery in disease control, such as in the case of locally (primary site) or regionally (cervical lymph nodes) advanced neoplasms of the oral cavity or in the case of neoplasms of the oral cavity

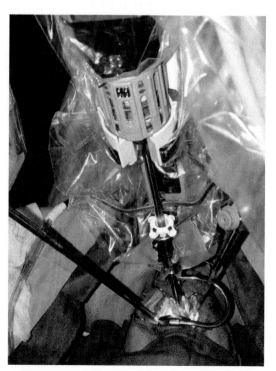

Fig. 3. Intraoperative photograph with oral retractors in place and arms of da Vinci robot within the surgical field.

that invade critical structures, such as the carotid artery, skull base, orbital cavity, and the intracranial cavity, thus hindering the ability to achieve adequate disease control through surgery. The extirpation of oral cancer can vary from minimally invasive procedures that require a short anesthetic exposure and hospitalization (**Fig. 4**) to procedures that can involve significant operations that encompass different body parts and a prolonged hospitalization and recovery process (**Fig. 5**). Furthermore, the overall health of the patient to withstand a major operation has to be considered when assessing the candidacy of a patient for surgical management of their oral cancer, irrespective of the resectability of their tumor due to the high risk for bleeding and airway compromise, because the surgical management of oral cancer will almost always require general anesthesia. Furthermore, aside from the critical anatomic structures and overall patient health, at the present time, there is no role for surgery in patients with distant metastatic disease; therefore, distant metastatic disease must be ruled out before proceeding with the surgical management of oral cancer. The only role of surgery for cases of metastatic cancer is securing the airway, if necessary, for a tracheostomy procedure or placement of long-term enteral nutrition access via a gastrostomy tube.

In this article, the authors discuss the role of surgery and techniques used today in the extirpation of malignant neoplasms of the oral cavity. The aim is for the reader to gain insight to the operative procedures and their indications and contraindications, and the decision-making process that goes into identifying which surgical technique to use in balancing optimal disease control and function/cosmesis.

SURGICAL MANAGEMENT OF THE PRIMARY TUMOR SITE
Margin Status

Of malignant neoplasms of the oral cavity, 90% are SCC. Excluding the lip, traditionally a 1- to 1.5-cm (10–15 mm) resection margin is recommended (**Fig. 6**). Obtaining a tumor-free surgical margin is critical from a locoregional disease control perspective and an overall survival perspective.[6] Therefore, following tumor extirpation, a critical parameter analyzed in the final pathologic report is the "margin status." Today, a negative (clear) margin is a margin where the invasive tumor is at least 5 mm away from the resected margin, and a close margin is a margin where the invasive tumor

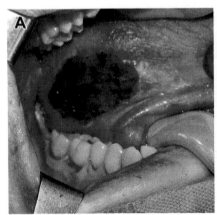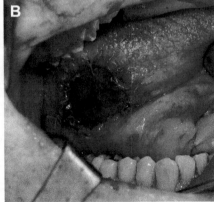

Fig. 4. (A, B) Intraoperative photograph following excision of premalignant lesion of the tongue, with reconstruction with an off-the-shelf porcine-derived construct.

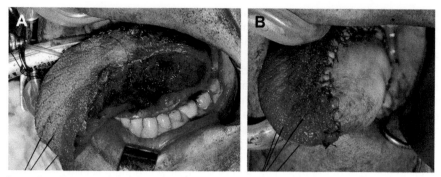

Fig. 5. (A, B) Intraoperative photograph following left oral hemiglossectomy with reconstruction of tongue with a fasciocutaneous radial forearm free flap.

is within 1 to 5 mm from the resected margin, and a positive (involved) margin is one that is less than 1 mm from the resected margin to the invasive tumor.[6] Controversy exists as to what constitutes an involved (positive), close, or clear (negative) margin, because a recent survey of head and neck surgeons found that 63% of respondents defined a close margin as a distance of less than 5 mm between the resection margin and invasive tumor, and a clear margin being a distance of 5 mm or greater between the 2.[7] A positive margin is considered an indication for adjuvant CTR or re-resection, whereas a close margin is an indication for adjuvant XRT.[8] Therefore, in cases of early-stage (T1 and T2) oral SCC with negative resection margins, in the absence of any adverse histologic features, the patient can be spared adjuvant therapy. Furthermore, the presence of a close (1–5 mm) margin has been demonstrated in several studies in decreasing overall survival and disease-free survival; therefore, additional adjuvant XRT is recommended.[6] Of the oral cavity subsites, lip cancers, in general, have the most favorable prognosis.[9] Lip cancer margins are the most conservative of all the oral cavity subsites, which are 0.5 to 1 cm (5–10 mm).

Tumor Extirpation Techniques

Glossectomy (tongue resection) is defined by the extent of tissue removed and the involved portion of the tongue (oral tongue vs base of tongue). Removal of less than

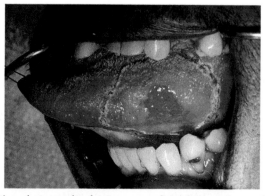

Fig. 6. Intraoperative photograph of 1.5-cm superficial (mucosal) margin marked out circumferentially using electrocautery.

one-third of the tongue is defined as a partial glossectomy; one-third to one-half is defined as a hemiglossectomy; one-half to three-quarters is defined as a subtotal glossectomy, and greater than three-quarters is defined as a total glossectomy (**Fig. 7**).

Removal of tumors that abut or invade the mandible or maxilla will require partial or complete removal of a small or large segment of bone in order to obtain clear surgical margins. In the case of the mandible, marginal mandibulectomy is a technique that involves removal of either a portion of the alveolar bone while maintaining the integrity of the inferior border of the mandible, versus removal of a portion of the inferior border of the mandible while preserving the integrity of the alveolus of the mandible. This technique is contraindicated in patients with a history of head and neck XRT where the mandible was part of the treatment field or in cases where there is clinical or radiographic invasion of the bone marrow of the mandible. This technique can weaken the structure of the mandible, and the general rule is if the mandible has 1 cm or less of the inferior border following tumor extirpation, then it must be reinforced with a mandibular reconstruction plate in order to reduce the risk for a pathologic fracture. In the case of lesions that abut or invade the maxilla, a maxillectomy procedure is performed. This procedure has various classification schemas that are based on the vertical and horizontal extent of the bony defect of the maxilla and the involvement of the nasal cavity or orbit.[10-13]

SCC of the buccal mucosa is considered a high-risk (aggressive) oral cancer subsite; therefore, multimodality therapy beginning with primary surgery followed by adjuvant therapy is the preferred recommendation for patients.[14,15] Surgery will consist of wide excision of the lesion with 1.0- to 1.5-cm mucosal and deep margins (**Fig. 8**). Furthermore, in cases where the lesion is in close proximity to the maxilla or mandible, consideration for maxillectomy (infrastructure, subtotal, or total) or mandibulectomy (marginal or segmental) should be considered. In locally advanced cases of buccal SCC, it is not uncommon to have to resect a portion or a segment of the maxilla and mandible as well as overlying skin, creating a complex through-and-through orofacial defect.

ROLE OF NECK DISSECTION (CERVICAL LYMPHADENECTOMY)

Cervical lymphadenectomy is the process of systematic removal of groups of lymph nodes within the neck for staging of cancer, decreasing disease burden, or guiding

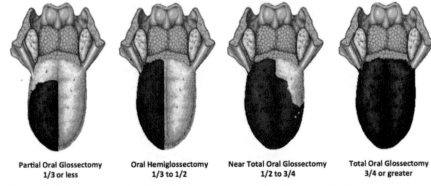

Partial Oral Glossectomy
1/3 or less

Oral Hemiglossectomy
1/3 to 1/2

Near Total Oral Glossectomy
1/2 to 3/4

Total Oral Glossectomy
3/4 or greater

Fig. 7. Oral glossectomy classification based on extent of tissue excised.

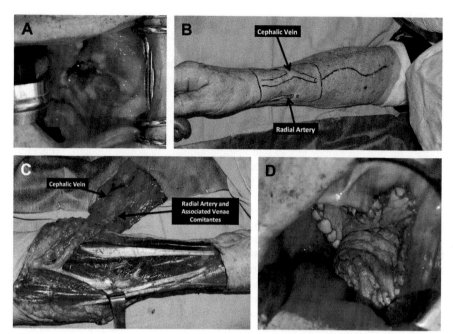

Fig. 8. (*A, C*) T3 SCC of the left buccal mucosa. (*B, C*) Marked out radial forearm free flap, which is commonly performed to reconstruct large defects of the cheek. (*D*) Free flap inset to reconstruct the postoncologic defect.

oncologic decision making. At the time of initial presentation, ~40% of patients will present with cancer metastasis to cervical lymph nodes.[16,17] Neck dissection is described as either elective or therapeutic. Elective neck dissection is performed in the case where no clinical or radiographic lymphadenopathy is noted, and removal of certain levels of lymph nodes is aimed at ruling out the presence of metastatic lymph nodes, which is critical in the decision-making process for adjuvant therapy and cancer outcome prognostication.[16] Therapeutic neck dissection is performed in the presence of either clinical or radiographic lymphadenopathy with the goal of determining the degree of disease burden and also the presence of extracapsular extension, which are indications for adjuvant XRT as well as chemotherapy.[16,18] The status of the cervical lymph nodes is considered the single most important prognosticator for oral cancer, because having a single metastatic lymph node will reduce 5-year survival by 50%.[16]

The role of elective neck dissection, that is, a neck dissection in the absence of clinical or radiographic evidence of cervical lymph node metastasis (also known as "N0" neck), has been debated for several decades. In 2015, a landmark prospective, randomized, controlled trial was published in the *New England Journal of Medicine* and provided evidence for the benefit of elective nodal dissection in cases of node-negative oral cancer.[19] However, at the present time, depending on institutional preference, a 3-mm depth of invasion is used as a cutoff for recommending a neck dissection in the N0 neck. Although a plethora of literature has been devoted to determining the ideal depth of invasion threshold for recommending a neck dissection in N0 patients or if all patients with invasive SCC should undergo a neck dissection, this decision is largely left to the patient after counseling the patient on the benefits of the elective neck dissection from an oncologic perspective versus the added morbidity from a neck dissection.

The neck dissection of oral and head and neck cancer dates back to 1906 with its initial description by Dr George Crile from the Cleveland Clinic in Ohio.[20,21] Dr Hayes Martin from Memorial Hospital in New York City would expand on the work of Dr Crile with his publication in 1951 that reviewed his experience in performing 1450 neck dissections.[21–23] The seminal work by Shah and colleagues[24–27] stratified the lymph nodes of the neck into the following lymph node groups: Ia (submental), Ib (submandibular), IIa and IIb (upper jugular), III (middle jugular), IV (lower jugular), Va and Vb (posterior triangle), VI (central compartment), and VII (superior mediastinal) (refer to **fig. 4** in Mel Mupparapu and Rabie M. Shanti's article, "Evaluation and Staging of Oral Cancer," in this issue). Of note, levels IIa and IIb are separated by the spinal accessory nerve (cranial nerve XI). The neck dissection in the ensuing decades would undergo several iterations and today is simply stratified based on the dissected lymph node groups or excised adjacent structures.[16] The modified radical neck dissection refers to cases where dissection removes lymph node levels I–V with removal of any of the following structures: spinal accessory nerve, internal jugular vein, and sternocleidomastoid muscle. If levels I–V lymph nodes are removed including all 3 of these structures, this is referred to as a radical neck dissection. If additional nonlymphatic (ie, neurovascular, muscular, or cutaneous) structures are excised such as the hypoglossal nerve, vagus nerve, carotid artery, paraspinal muscles, or overlying skin of the neck, this is referred to as an extended radical neck dissection.[16] Today, such extensive neck dissections are infrequently performed in the primary setting, and more commonly, a functional type of neck dissection is performed. The functional types of neck dissection includes the selective neck dissection (levels I–IV) or supraomohyoid neck dissection (levels I–III) with preservation of all the aforementioned nonlymphatic structures. This is performed through conservative cutaneous incisions in order to reduce the morbidity and improve the cosmesis of the overall outcome of the patient (**Fig. 9**).

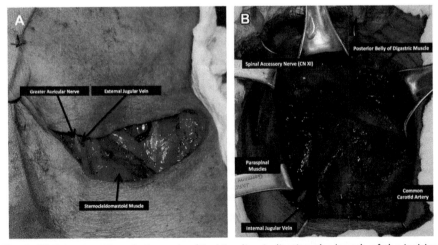

Fig. 9. (*A*) Intraoperative photograph of incision line indicating the length of the incision performed at the authors' institution. (*B*) Intraoperative photograph of critical structures that are dissected during a neck dissection.

SUMMARY

Over the past 4 decades, a plethora of advancements have been made in the management of head and neck cancers, including advancements in diagnostic (ie, PET/ computed tomography) and nonsurgical treatment modalities, such as intensity modulated radiation therapy, proton therapy, targeted systemic therapy (ie, Cetuximab), and most recently, immunotherapy. Furthermore, a move toward minimally invasive surgical procedures has occurred with the reduction of the extent of a neck dissection being performed and also ground-breaking advancements such as TORS. Nonetheless, oral cancers are primarily managed with surgery as a primary treatment modality; therefore, familiarity of the types of extirpative procedures and the rationale for their use is imperative for the practitioner involved in the care of patients with oral cancer.

REFERENCES

1. Department of Veterans Affairs Laryngeal Cancer Study Group, Wolf GT, Fisher SG, Hong WK, et al. Induction chemotherapy plus radiation compared with surgery plus radiation in patients with advanced laryngeal cancer. N Engl J Med 1991;324(24):1685–90.
2. Esteller E, Vega MC, Lopez M, et al. Salvage surgery after locoregional failure in head and neck carcinoma patients treated with chemoradiotherapy. Eur Arch Otorhinolaryngol 2011;268(2):295–301.
3. Leon X, Quer M, Orus C, et al. Results of salvage surgery for local or regional recurrence after larynx preservation with induction chemotherapy and radiotherapy. Head Neck 2001;23(9):733–8.
4. Kao SS, Micklem J, Ofo E, et al. A comparison of oncological outcomes between transoral surgical and non-surgical treatment protocols in the management of oropharyngeal squamous cell carcinoma. J Laryngol Otol 2017;1–7 [Epub ahead of print].
5. Hockstein NG, O'Malley BW Jr, Weinstein GS. Assessment of intraoperative safety in transoral robotic surgery. Laryngoscope 2006;116(2):165–8.
6. Dillon JK, Brown CB, McDonald TM, et al. How does the close surgical margin impact recurrence and survival when treating oral squamous cell carcinoma? J Oral Maxillofac Surg 2015;73(6):1182–8.
7. Tasche KK, Buchakjian MR, Pagedar NA, et al. Definition of "close margin" in oral cancer surgery and association of margin distance with local recurrence rate. JAMA Otolaryngol Head Neck Surg 2017. [Epub ahead of print].
8. Cooper JS, Pajak TF, Forastiere AA, et al. Postoperative concurrent radiotherapy and chemotherapy for high-risk squamous-cell carcinoma of the head and neck. N Engl J Med 2004;350(19):1937–44.
9. Biasoli ER, Valente VB, Mantovan B, et al. Lip cancer: a clinicopathological study and treatment outcomes in a 25-year experience. J Oral Maxillofac Surg 2016; 74(7):1360–7.
10. Brown JS, Rogers SN, McNally DN, et al. A modified classification for the maxillectomy defect. Head Neck 2000;22(1):17–26.
11. Okay DJ, Genden E, Buchbinder D, et al. Prosthodontic guidelines for surgical reconstruction of the maxilla: a classification system of defects. J Prosthet Dent 2001;86(4):352–63.
12. Cordeiro PG, Chen CM. A 15-year review of midface reconstruction after total and subtotal maxillectomy: part II. Technical modifications to maximize aesthetic and functional outcomes. Plast Reconstr Surg 2012;129(1):139–47.

13. Cordeiro PG, Chen CM. A 15-year review of midface reconstruction after total and subtotal maxillectomy: part I. Algorithm and outcomes. Plast Reconstr Surg 2012; 129(1):124–36.

14. Lin CS, Jen YM, Kao WY, et al. Improved outcomes in buccal squamous cell carcinoma. Head Neck 2013;35(1):65–71.

15. Lin CS, Jen YM, Cheng MF, et al. Squamous cell carcinoma of the buccal mucosa: an aggressive cancer requiring multimodality treatment. Head Neck 2006;28(2):150–7.

16. Holmes JD. Neck dissection: nomenclature, classification, and technique. Oral Maxillofac Surg Clin North Am 2008;20(3):459–75.

17. Mendenhall WM, Million RR, Cassisi NJ. Elective neck irradiation in squamous-cell carcinoma of the head and neck. Head Neck Surg 1980;3(1):15–20.

18. Shetty AV, Wong DJ. Systemic treatment for squamous cell carcinoma of the head and neck. Otolaryngol Clin North Am 2017;50(4):775–82.

19. D'Cruz AK, Vaish R, Kapre N, et al. Elective versus therapeutic neck dissection in node-negative oral cancer. N Engl J Med 2015;373(6):521–9.

20. Crile G. III. On the technique of operations upon the head and neck. Ann Surg 1906;44(6):842–50.

21. Carlson ER, Cheung A, Smith B, et al. Neck dissections for oral/head and neck cancer: 1906-2006. J Oral Maxillofac Surg 2006;64(1):4–11.

22. Martin H. The case for prophylactic neck dissection. Cancer 1951;4(1):92–7.

23. Martin H, Del Valle B, Ehrlich H, et al. Neck dissection. Cancer 1951;4(3):441–99.

24. Candela FC, Kothari K, Shah JP. Patterns of cervical node metastases from squamous carcinoma of the oropharynx and hypopharynx. Head Neck 1990;12(3): 197–203.

25. Candela FC, Shah J, Jaques DP, et al. Patterns of cervical node metastases from squamous carcinoma of the larynx. Arch Otolaryngol Head Neck Surg 1990; 116(4):432–5.

26. Shah JP, Candela FC, Poddar AK. The patterns of cervical lymph node metastases from squamous carcinoma of the oral cavity. Cancer 1990;66(1):109–13.

27. Shah JP. Patterns of cervical lymph node metastasis from squamous carcinomas of the upper aerodigestive tract. Am J Surg 1990;160(4):405–9.

Chemotherapy for Oral Cancer

Lee Hartner, MD

KEYWORDS

- Chemotherapy • Oral cancer • Chemoradiation • Cisplatin • Cetuximab
- Nivolumab • Pembrolizumab

KEY POINTS

- Adjuvant chemotherapy has not been shown to improve treatment outcomes in patients with oral cancer after surgery and should not be used.
- Adjuvant combined chemotherapy and radiation improves survival for patients with extracapsular extension in nodal metastases and positive resection margins. Cisplatin should be used.
- Patients with oral cancer can be treated with primary chemoradiation, although the impact on survival is unclear. Cisplatin is the standard agent to combine with radiation. Cetuximab has not been well-studied.
- Induction chemotherapy can be used selectively, but its impact on overall survival remains unclear and is associated with significant toxicity.
- Anti– programmed cell death-ligand 1 antibodies have been shown to improve survival for patients with metastatic disease after treatment with platinum-based chemotherapy.

INTRODUCTION

The past several years have seen major advances in the use of systemic therapy for treatment of patients with oral cancer. Systemic therapy refers to chemotherapy and immunotherapy drugs, which are playing an increasingly important role in treatment. Chemotherapy has classically been used either as a primary treatment modality or in combination with radiation, where it is used as a radiation sensitizer. Based on the results of pivotal trials during the past decade, the use of systemic therapy has expanded in scope and has resulted in meaningful improvements in patient outcomes. This article discusses the different uses for systemic therapy in the treatment of patients with oral squamous cell carcinoma and reviews the current state of practice and areas of future investigation. In discussing studies, the relevance to patients with oral cancer are highlighted. It is important to remember that studies in patients

Conflicts of Interest: None to report.
Abramson Cancer Center at Pennsylvania Hospital, 230 West Washington Square, Philadelphia, PA 19106, USA
E-mail address: Lee.Hartner@uphs.upenn.edu

Dent Clin N Am 62 (2018) 87–97
http://dx.doi.org/10.1016/j.cden.2017.08.006

with squamous cell carcinoma of the head and neck include patients with different primary sites and they are not always represented in the same relative amounts. Despite that, however, the results of these studies are in most cases applied to patients with primary tumors of all different subsites.

ADJUVANT CHEMOTHERAPY

The primary treatment modality for patients with oral cancer is surgery when possible without undue morbidity. Adjuvant chemotherapy is given after surgery in many types of cancer for reducing the incidence of metastatic recurrence. At the present time, adjuvant chemotherapy has no established role in the treatment of patients after surgery for oral cancer. The most recent update of a very large metaanalysis examining the role of chemotherapy in treatment of patients with head and neck cancer found no evidence of benefit.[1] It included a total of 2567 patients taken from 6 studies that included patients with oral cancer. Therefore, adjuvant chemotherapy should only be used in the context of a clinical trial.

ADJUVANT CHEMORADIOTHERAPY

In addition to studies of chemotherapy as a standalone adjuvant treatment modality, multiple studies have examined the use of concurrent chemotherapy and radiation. In this setting, chemotherapy is given as a radiation sensitizer with the goal of reducing radiation resistance. Multiple studies have found this approach is superior to radiation alone in patients with an increased risk of recurrence. The 2 largest trials examining this question, unfortunately, came to different conclusions. In the EORTC trial 22,931, a total of 334 patients were treated with either radiation alone or radiation combined with cisplatin 100 mg/m^2 given on days 1, 22, and 43.[2] The same treatments were compared in RTOG 9501, which enrolled a total of 459 patients.[3,4] However, these 2 studies had different enrollment criteria, defining high-risk disease differently (**Table 1**). As a result, they unfortunately came to different conclusions regarding the benefit of adjuvant chemoradiation. Based on analysis of these 2 studies, adjuvant chemoradiation seems to improve outcomes in patients with extracapsular extension

Table 1 Adjuvant chemoradiation: comparison between EORTC 22931 and RTOG 9501		
	EORTC 22931	**RTOG 9501**
Number of patients	334	459
Oral cavity patients	87	112
Stage	pT3 or pT4/any N or pT1 or pT2/N2 or N3	Any T stage, N2b or higher N stage
Unfavorable pathologic findings	ECE, positive margins, PNI, VTE	2 or more positive nodes, ECE, positive margins
Radiation	54 Gy with boost to 66 Gy	60 Gy with boost to 66 Gy
Chemotherapy	Cisplatin 100 mg/m^2 days 1, 22, and 43	Cisplatin 100 mg/m^2 days 1, 22, and 43
Findings	Improved 5 y PFS and OS	Improved DFS only for ECE, positive margins

Abbreviations: ECE, extracapsular extension; OS, overall survival; PFS, progression-free survival; PNI, perineural invasion; VTE, vascular tumor embolism.
    Data from Refs.[2-4]

of nodal metastases and in those with positive resection margins. Both studies included a sizable population of patients with oral cancer, approximately 25% to 30% of enrollment in both. Therefore, these findings can be reasonably applied to patients with resected oral cancers. No definitive evidence exists supporting improvement in outcomes for patients with any other high-risk features, including vascular invasion, perineural invasion, T3 and T4 pathologic stage or involvement of 2 or more lymph nodes. Current consensus treatment guidelines recommend that the use of chemoradiation be considered on a case-by-case basis for patients with 1 or more high-risk features other than extracapsular extension of nodal metastases or positive margins.[5]

For patients who are candidates for combined chemotherapy and radiation, there is no clear consensus on choice of chemotherapy regimen. Both randomized studies addressing this issue used cisplatin 100 mg/m^2 on days 1, 22, and 43. However, high-dose cisplatin, although the only regimen supported by randomized phase III clinical trials, is associated with significant risk for acute and late toxicities. Significant risks include kidney failure, hearing loss, tinnitus, nausea, vomiting, and peripheral neuropathy. Furthermore, data clearly indicate that radiation complications (both acute and chronic) are more common in patients treated with chemotherapy. Because of these issues, there has been considerable interest in alternatives to high-dose cisplatin. In the RTOG 9501 trial, only 125 patients (61%) could complete all 3 cycles of cisplatin. Forty-seven patients (23%) only received 2 cycles. In a subset analysis, the 2-year locoregional control rate was 82% in the group that received all planned chemotherapy or had a minor variation in treatment, which was the same as that found for the study as a whole.[3] Some have used this as justification for giving only 2 cycles of high-dose cisplatin, although this question has not been studied in a prospective randomized trial. The use of lower dose cisplatin has also been studied with some evidence of benefit compared with radiation alone.[6,7] Although no prospective randomized trial has been completed comparing high-dose cisplatin with lower dose weekly cisplatin (typically given at a dose of 30–40 mg/m^2) in the adjuvant chemoradiation setting, the currently available evidence suggests that it has similar efficacy and less acute toxicity.[8] It is currently a widely used alternative to high-dose cisplatin despite the lack of supporting phase III data. As discussed elsewhere in this article, 1 phase III trial that examined patients being treated with definitive chemoradiation (patients who were not candidates for surgery) found that use of high-dose cisplatin significantly reduced the risk of local recurrence. Based on this and lack of a phase III trial in the adjuvant chemoradiation setting, high-dose cisplatin should be used unless there is a medical contraindication.

Cetuximab, a monoclonal antibody directed against the epidermal growth factor receptor, has an established role in the primary treatment of locally advanced unresectable oral cancer when given in combination with radiation, but it has not been studied in the adjuvant setting in combination with radiation. This agent, as well as the chemotherapy agent docetaxel given on a weekly schedule, remain under active investigation, both separately and in combination. However, they are not currently considered standard treatment options for use with adjuvant chemoradiation.

PRIMARY CHEMORADIATION

Surgery is often recommended for the initial management of patients with early stage oral squamous cell carcinoma, but many patients present with locally advanced disease that precludes resection. This is a common occurrence in cancers of other subsites as well. The use of combined chemotherapy and radiation has been studied extensively for the treatment of locally advanced oral and other head and neck cancers, both as a means of organ preservation and as a primary therapy, even when organ preservation is not necessarily a goal. Notably, although oral cancers were well-represented in trials of adjuvant chemoradiation, they have typically been underrepresented in trials of primary chemoradiation.

The initial study detailing the benefits of primary concurrent chemoradiation was the VA Larynx trial, although this study used initial chemotherapy followed by combined chemotherapy and radiation in responding patients.[9] This study was the first to show that the addition of chemotherapy (cisplatin and 5-fluoracil [5-FU] in this study) to radiation could improve organ preservation. Forastiere and colleagues[10] subsequently confirmed the benefit of combined chemotherapy and radiation in larynx cancer. Although this study found no differences in survival between patients treated with induction chemotherapy followed by radiation versus chemoradiation versus radiation alone, it did find a significantly improved organ preservation rate associated with chemoradiation (88% vs 75% for induction chemotherapy and 70% for radiation alone). Along with these trials, multiple other studies have been done, most in patients with either laryngeal or oropharyngeal squamous cell carcinoma. According to the most updated report of the Meta-Analysis of Chemotherapy on Head and Neck Cancer, published in 2009, the use of chemotherapy in addition to definitive local therapy (in this case, radiation) improved survival with an absolute benefit of 6.5% in 5-year survival.[1] Notably, no benefit was seen in patients older than 70 years and similar benefit was seen for all subsites, including oral. Also, supporting the usefulness of primary chemoradiation was a single-institution series from the University of Chicago that examined 111 patients, all with oral squamous cell carcinoma, treated at their institution from 1994 to 2008. They found no difference in overall or progression-free survival between patients treated with surgery first and those treated with primary chemoradiation.[11]

Initial studies of primary chemoradiation used high-dose cisplatin in the same manner that it was used in the adjuvant chemoradiation trials and, as in those studies, toxicity associated with 3 cycles of high-dose cisplatin was significant. Although the efficacy of 2 cycles of high-dose cisplatin versus 3 cycles has not been studied in a prospective manner in the adjuvant setting, it has been examined in one study in the primary treatment setting. In RTOG 0129, chemoradiation with conventional fractionation and 3 cycles of cisplatin 100 mg/m^2 was compared with chemoradiation with accelerated boost radiation (42 fractions given over 6 weeks) and only 2 cycles of cisplatin 100 mg/m^2.[12] This study found no difference in overall survival between these 2 groups, although this does not definitively establish that 2 cycles of cisplatin are equivalent to 3, because 2 variables were changed between the groups. Also, similar to the adjuvant therapy setting, multiple studies have examined use of lower dose weekly cisplatin (typically 30–40 mg/m^2).[13,14] These studies have found that the use of weekly cisplatin is safe and effective compared with radiotherapy alone. One study has compared high-dose cisplatin with weekly cisplatin given at a dose of 30 mg/m^2. This study, which enrolled mostly patients with oral cancer not amenable to surgery, found that use of high-dose cisplatin every 3 weeks was associated with a 42% reduction in the risk of local recurrence.[15] Based on these data, high-dose cisplatin is preferred over weekly cisplatin, and weekly cisplatin should be reserved for patients who are not able to be treated with high-dose cisplatin because of medical contraindications. Although it has not been compared directly with high-dose cisplatin, at the present time, lower dose cisplatin is considered an appropriate treatment option based on these data.

Cetuximab has also been studied in combination with radiation for the primary treatment of locally advanced squamous cell carcinoma of the head and neck. In a pivotal trial, a total of 424 patients with cancers of the larynx, oropharynx, and hypopharynx, treatment with radiation alone was compared with treatment with radiation plus cetuximab.[16] In this study, cetuximab was given weekly, with an initial loading dose of 400 mg/m^2 1 week before the start of radiotherapy, followed by 250 mg/m^2 weekly during radiation treatment. At a median follow-up of 54 months, there was a significant improvement in overall survival observed in the group treated with cetuximab (median of 49.0 months vs 29.3 months). Of note, this study did not include patients with oral cancer, so conclusions cannot be drawn regarding the efficacy of cetuximab combined with radiation for treatment of oral cancer at this time. Also of importance, patients older than 65 years and those with poorer performance status did not clearly benefit.

Based on the data summarized, it is most reasonable to conclude that primary chemoradiation has a definite role in the management of unresectable oral squamous cell carcinoma. Compared with radiation alone, it improves survival and reduces the risk of recurrence. However, it does not seem to benefit patients older than 70 years. Use of high-dose cisplatin is preferred for fit patients. For patients not appropriate for high-dose cisplatin, lower dose weekly regimens are recommended. Cetuximab, although used in this setting, is not supported by any data in patients with oral cancer and cannot be recommended routinely.

INDUCTION CHEMOTHERAPY

Induction chemotherapy refers to initial chemotherapy treatment before definitive local therapy. This treatment typically is combination chemotherapy, and the use of such treatment has some putative advantages. These advantages include potentially reducing the risk of metastatic recurrence and downsizing of the primary tumor to improve locoregional control. One of the first uses of induction chemotherapy was in the VA Larynx trial.[9] In that study, patients were treated with 2 cycles of full-dose cisplatin and 5-FU before going on to treatment with definitive local therapy based on response. More recent studies have combined induction chemotherapy with primary chemoradiation, in an effort to both improve locoregional control and decrease metastatic recurrence. Those studies have also studied the addition of other agents to cisplatin and 5-FU, most importantly docetaxel. For example, in the TAX 324 trial (A Randomized Phase III Multicenter Trial of Neoadjuvant Docetaxel (Taxotere) Plus Cisplatin Plus 5-Fluorouracil Versus Neoadjuvant Cisplatin Plus 5-Fluorouracil in Patients With Locally Advanced Inoperable Squamous Cell Carcinoma of the Head and Neck), induction treatment with cisplatin and 5-FU was compared with TPF (docetaxel 75 mg/m^2, cisplatin 100 mg/m^2, and 5-FU 1000 mg/m^2 continuous infusion on days 1–5).[17] This study enrolled 501 patients, and after 3 cycles of induction chemotherapy, all patients were treated with radiation combined with carboplatin. At a median follow-up of 72 months, the TPF regimen was associated with an improvement in overall survival as well as progression-free survival. In EORTC 24971/TAX 323, a slightly different TPF regimen (cisplatin 75 mg/m^2 and 5-FU 750 mg/m^2 continuous infused on days 1–4) was used, and in this study, TPF also improved progression-free survival and overall survival.[18] This study did not use chemoradiation after induction therapy. Rather, patients were treated with radiation alone. Both studies included patients with oral cancers, about 13% to 17% of the study population. Although those 2 regimens have not been compared directly, either is an acceptable induction chemotherapy regimen. Notably, use of high-dose cisplatin combined with radiation after treatment with full-dose induction chemotherapy is not recommended owing to significant safety concerns.

The improvement in survival observed with the addition of docetaxel to cisplatin and 5-FU induction chemotherapy raised important questions regarding the optimal use of TPF induction chemotherapy. Although it had been shown to improve survival compared with cisplatin and 5-FU, it was also associated with a significant increase in toxicity, including some treatment-related deaths. In addition, it remained unclear whether the combination of TPF with chemoradiation could improve outcomes compared with use of chemoradiation alone. Multiple studies have since been initiated to answer this important question. In the DeCIDE trial (A phase III randomized trial of docetaxel, cisplatin, 5-fluorouracil, (TPF) induction chemotherapy in patients with N2/N3 locally advanced squamous cell carcinoma of the head and neck), 280 patients with N2 or N3 disease were treated with either upfront chemoradiation or 2 cycles of TPF followed by chemoradiation using docetaxel, 5-FU, and hydroxyurea.[19] This study enrolled only 280 and, thus far, has found no significant difference in outcome between these 2 groups. Also relevant is a phase II/III trial centered in Italy that enrolled 421 patients and which has only been reported in abstract form.[20] Treatment in this study was 3 cycles of TPF induction chemotherapy followed by chemoradiation compared with treatment with chemoradiation alone. This study also included a second randomization between PF (cisplatin, 5-FU) and cetuximab-based chemoradiation. At a median follow-up of 41 months, treatment with induction chemotherapy significantly improved overall survival compared with concurrent chemoradiation alone. Median survival was 54 versus 30 months, with 3-year survival rates of 58% versus 46%.

At the present time, therefore, the use of induction chemotherapy with TPF followed by chemoradiation remains of unclear benefit compared with chemoradiation alone. Studies have shown that, although it is superior to PF-based induction chemotherapy, it is not definitely superior to treatment with modern chemoradiation without induction. Also, as noted, it is associated with a significant incidence of both hematologic and nonhematologic toxicity. Therefore, although induction chemotherapy can be considered in selected patients, it is not yet a routine standard treatment option. The actual efficacy in oral cancers also remains somewhat poorly defined. Although patients with oral cancer were represented in the TPF versus PF trials and were also included in the DeCIDE trial at a rate similar to those studies, the degree of their representation in the Italian trial is not known. Further study is needed to define more clearly the role of induction chemotherapy in patients with locally advanced oral cancers.

METASTATIC DISEASE

The treatment of metastatic oral squamous cell carcinoma has changed significantly over the past several years. Although metastatic disease is an uncommon occurrence in patients, classically, treatment options have been limited and responses not common. However, recent studies have identified new agents that have been shown to improve survival outcomes in the metastatic disease setting. Treatment of patients with metastatic disease is palliative and the median survival of patients with metastatic oral cancer mirrors that of patients with head and neck cancer in general, which is approximately 6 to 12 months.[21]

Standard chemotherapy for front-line treatment of metastatic disease has typically been with cisplatin or carboplatin containing regimens. These drugs have activity as single agents, but in the front-line setting, they are most commonly used in combination with other chemotherapy agents, such as 5-FU, docetaxel, and paclitaxel. At the present time, there is no convincing evidence supporting any efficacy difference be-tween these 2 agents, although there are clear differences in side effects. Carboplatin is associated more commonly with myelosuppression than cisplatin and avoids the more significant cisplatin-related complications of neuropathy, hearing toxicity, and acute kidney injury. For these reasons, carboplatin is often used in the treatment of patients with metastatic disease. To date, there is no convincing evidence that use of a platinum-based combination chemotherapy regimen improves survival compared with use of single-agent chemotherapy, although the evidence does indicate that response rate is higher with combination therapy. For example, cisplatin with 5-FU has been found to have a response rate of about 30%, which is higher than cisplatin alone and about the same as cisplatin and paclitaxel.[22,23] In a study comparing cisplatin and 5-FU with cisplatin and paclitaxel, response rates were the same (27% vs 26%) and median overall survival was also the same (8.7 months vs 8.1 months).[22] In an older study that compared cisplatin, 5-FU, and the combination, there was again no difference in overall survival between these 3 groups at about 5.7 months for all three.[23]

Non–platinum-based chemotherapy has been studied in a limited fashion and has not been compared directly with platinum-based chemotherapy. For example, the combination of gemcitabine (3000 mg/m^2) and paclitaxel (150 mg/m^2) given every 14 days was studied in an Southwest Oncology Group phase II trial and found to have a response rate of 28% with an overall survival of about 8 months.[24] Whether these results are superior to those with single agent paclitaxel remains unanswered. Also, the combination of paclitaxel and cetuximab given weekly was found to have a response rate of 54% and an overall survival of 8.1 months.[25] For patients unable to tolerate platinum-based treatment, these are reasonable options.

In addition to its role as a radiation sensitizer for patients with locally advanced dis-ease, cetuximab has been studied in the treatment of metastatic disease. Early studies with this agent were done for the treatment of recurrent metastatic disease and, in those studies, it was used as a single agent with evidence of modest activity as discussed elsewhere in this article. To improve treatment outcomes in the first-line treatment setting, studies were done combining cetuximab with platinum-based combination chemotherapy regimens in previously untreated patients. In the phase III EXTREME trial (Erbitux in First-Line Treatment of Recurrent or Metastatic Head and Neck Cancer), 442 patients with recurrent or metastatic head and neck cancer were treated with platinum (either cisplatin or carboplatin) plus 5-FU with or without cetuximab.[26] Patients with oral cancer were well-represented in this study, accounting for about 20% of the treatment population. In this study, chemotherapy was given for a maximum of 6 cycles, after which cetuximab could be continued as a single agent. This study found that the addition of cetuximab resulted in a significant improvement in overall survival, increased from 7.4 months to 10.1 months. Both progression-free survival and response rate were also increased. This improvement came without a sig-nificant increase in severe toxicity, and based on this data, cetuximab has been approved by the US Food and Drug Administration for use in the front-line treatment setting in combination with platinum and 5-FU–based chemotherapy.

Panitumumab, a fully human monoclonal antibody also directed against the epidermal growth factor receptor, has been studied in the treatment of metastatic head and neck cancers. Currently, however, this agent does not have an established role in the treatment of head and neck cancer and has not been shown to improve sur-vival when given with front-line cisplatin plus 5-FU chemotherapy.[27]

For patients with progression after front-line chemotherapy, multiple options exist. These include cytotoxic chemotherapy, programmed cell death (PD)-1 inhibitors, cetuximab, and small molecule tyrosine kinase inhibitors. Choice of treatment depends on prior treatment history, performance status, and the presence or absence of significant medical comorbid illnesses. There has been considerable excitement surrounding use of PD-1 inhibitors, which have been found recently to improve survival in this treatment setting.

PD-1 is a receptor expressed on T cells, B cells, and natural killer cells. It functions, along with PD-ligand 1 (PD-L1) and PD-L2, to suppress immune function by downregulating the activity of effector T cells. PD-L1 and PD-L2 are expressed on many different cell types throughout the body and they are also expressed commonly on tumor cells. By taking advantage of this receptor–ligand complex, tumor cells can evade destruction by effector T cells. Many different monoclonal antibodies have been developed for the purpose of interfering with the PD-1/PD-L1 axis. These agents do not cause side effects commonly associated with chemotherapy, such as myelosuppression, nausea, vomiting, and fatigue. However, they can cause a variety of autoimmune toxicities, and although they are often well-tolerated as single agents, toxicity can occur suddenly and be severe, even potentially fatal, if not recognized and treated promptly. Common side effects include rash, diarrhea, hepatitis, thyroiditis, hypophysitis, and pneumonitis. Approved agents to date include nivolumab, pembrolizumab, and atezolizumab. Both nivolumab and pembrolizumab have shown activity in the treatment of recurrent and metastatic head and neck cancers and both are currently FDA approved for the treatment of metastatic head and neck cancer with progression after first-line platinum-containing chemotherapy.

Nivolumab was studied in a phase III clinical trial that enrolled patients with platinum-refractory recurrent or metastatic disease. Notably, about one-half of the enrolled patients had metastatic oral cancers. It was compared with investigator's choice of single-agent therapy, with options including cetuximab, methotrexate, and docetaxel.[28] In this study, a total of 361 patients were treated and nivolumab improved overall survival from 5.1 months to 7.5 months. PD-L1 expression was measured in all patients, and it was found that, in patients with expression of 1% or higher, survival was improved with the use of nivolumab. The FDA approval of nivolumab does not require measurement of PD-L1 expression. It is given at a dose of 3 mg/kg intravenously every 2 weeks.

Pembrolizumab, in contrast, was approved provisionally in August 2016 based on the results of a phase Ib clinical trial.[29] This study enrolled 174 patients with progression on or after platinum-based chemotherapy. Initial results were notable for a 16% response rate, notably including 8 complete responses (5% of the population). Also, most responses (23 of 28) lasted longer than 6 months. Updated results presented in 2016 at the American Society of Clinical Oncology meeting were notable for median overall survival of 8 months and 12-month survival of 38%.[30] This agent is currently FDA approved at a fixed dose of 200 mg given intravenously every 3 weeks, and also does not require measurement of tumor PD-L1 expression. Two phase III trials are ongoing to confirm these results.

In addition to these monoclonal antibodies, cetuximab has modest activity in the treatment of recurrent or metastatic head and neck cancers. For example, in 1 series of 103 patients who had progression after previous treatment with platinum-based chemotherapy, it was associated with a response rate of 13% and a median survival of 7.5 months.[31]

Multiple small molecule tyrosine kinase inhibitors have been studied in the treatment of advanced head and neck cancer. These include gefitnib,[32,33] afatinib,[34] sunitinib,[35] and erlotinib.[36] To date, however, no study has found evidence of convincing activity or improvement in overall survival associated with these agents.

Various cytotoxic chemotherapy drugs have been studied in the second-line setting and beyond. Overall, studies have failed to document significant benefit and, to date, there is no study that has found evidence of improved survival associated with cytotoxic chemotherapy in the second-line setting or beyond. Agents that have been studied include methotrexate,[33] gemcitabine,[37] paclitaxel,[38] docetaxel,[39] and 5-FU.[23] Choice of agent depends on prior treatment history and differences in expected toxicity between the agents, because there are no comparative studies to guide decision making.

Given the limited available treatment options for patients with metastatic disease, particularly after second-line treatment with PD-1 inhibitor–based therapy, it is important to closely monitor symptoms and to discuss prognosis and goals of care. Recurrent and metastatic head and neck cancer carries the potential for considerable morbidity combined with short survival, and a transition away from active treatment and toward comfort care and hospice should be pursued when appropriate.

REFERENCES

1. Pignon JP, le Maitre A, Maillard E, et al. Meta-analysis of chemotherapy in head and neck cancer (MACH-NC): an update on 93 randomised trials and 17,346 patients. Radiother Oncol 2009;92:4–14.
2. Bernier J, Domenge C, Ozsahin M, et al. Postoperative irradiation with or without concomitant chemotherapy for locally advanced head and neck cancer. N Engl J Med 2004;350:1945–52.
3. Cooper JS, Pajak TF, Forastiere AA, et al. Postoperative concurrent radiotherapy and chemotherapy for high-risk squamous-cell carcinoma of the head and neck. N Engl J Med 2004;350:1937–44.
4. Cooper JS, Zhang Q, Pajak TF, et al. Long-term follow-up of the RTOG 9501/intergroup phase III trial: postoperative concurrent radiation therapy and chemotherapy in high-risk squamous cell carcinoma of the head and neck. Int J Radiat Oncol Biol Phys 2012;84:1198–205.
5. Head and Neck Cancers. Version 1.2017. 2017. NCCN Guidelines. Available at: https://www.nccn.org/professionals/physician_gls/pdf/head-and-neck.pdf. Accessed April 12, 2017.
6. Bachaud JM, Cohen-Jonathan E, Alzieu C, et al. Combined postoperative radiotherapy and weekly cisplatin infusion for locally advanced head and neck carcinoma: final report of a randomized trial. Int J Radiat Oncol Biol Phys 1996;36:999–1004.
7. Franchin G, Minatel E, Politi D, et al. Postoperative reduced dose of cisplatin concomitant with radiation therapy in high- risk head and neck squamous cell carcinoma. Cancer 2009;115:2464–71.
8. Melotek JM, Cooper BT, Koshy M, et al. Weekly versus every-three weeks platinum-based chemoradiation regimens for head and neck cancer. J Otolaryngol Head Neck Surg 2016;45:62–70.
9. The Department of Veterans Affairs Laryngeal Cancer Study Group. Induction chemotherapy plus radiation compared with surgery plus radiation in patients with advanced laryngeal cancer. N Engl J Med 1991;324:1685–90.
10. Forastiere AA, Goepfert H, Maor M, et al. Concurrent chemotherapy and radiotherapy for organ preservation in advanced laryngeal cancer. N Engl J Med 2003;349:2091–8.
11. Stenson KM, Kunnavakkam R, Cohen EE, et al. Chemoradiation for patients with advanced oral cavity cancer. Laryngoscope 2010;120:93–9.

12. Nguyen-Tan PF, Zhang Q, Ang KK, et al. Randomized phase III trial to test accelerated versus standard fractionation in combination with concurrent cisplatin for head and neck carcinomas in the Radiation Therapy Oncology Group 0129 trial: long-term report of efficacy and toxicity. J Clin Oncol 2014;32:3858–66.

13. Sharma A, Mohanti BK, Thakar A, et al. Concomitant chemoradiation versus radical radiotherapy in advanced squamous cell carcinoma of oropharynx and nasopharynx using weekly cisplatin: a phase II randomized trial. Ann Oncol 2010;21:2272–7.

14. Traynor AM, Richards GM, Hartig GK, et al. Comprehensive IMRT plus weekly cisplatin for advanced head and neck cancer: the University of Wisconsin experience. Head Neck 2010;32:599–606.

15. Noronha V, Joshi A, Patil VM, et al. Phase III randomized trial comparing weekly versus three-weekly (W3W) cisplatin in patients receiving chemoradiation for locally advanced head and neck cancer. J Clin Oncol 2017;35(Suppl 15); abstr 6007.

16. Bonner JA, Harari PM, Giralt J, et al. Radiotherapy plus cetuximab for squamous-cell carcinoma of the head and neck. N Engl J Med 2006;354:567–78.

17. Lorch JH, Goloubeva O, Haddad RI, et al. Induction chemotherapy with cisplatin and fluorouracil alone or in combination with docetaxel in locally advanced squamous-cell cancer of the head and neck: long-term results of the TAX 324 randomised phase 3 trial. Lancet Oncol 2011;12:153–9.

18. Vermorken JB, Remenar E, van Herpen C, et al. Cisplatin, fluorouracil, and docetaxel in unresectable head and neck cancer. N Engl J Med 2007;357:1695–704.

19. Cohen EE, Karrison TG, Kocherginsky M, et al. Phase III randomized trial of induction chemotherapy in patients with N2 or N3 locally advanced head and neck cancer. J Clin Oncol 2014;32:2735–43.

20. Ghi MG, Paccagnella A, Ferrari D, et al. Concomitant chemoradiation (CRT) or cetuximab/RT (CET/RT) versus induction Docetaxel/Cisplatin/5-Fluorouracil (TPF) followed by CRT or CET/RT in patients with Locally Advanced Squamous Cell Carcinoma of Head and Neck (LASCCHN). A randomized phase III factorial study (NCT01086826). J Clin Oncol 2014;32(Suppl 15); abstr 6004.

21. Shah D, Hoffman GR. Outcome of head and neck cancer patients who did not receive curative-intent treatment. J Oral Maxillofac Surg 2017. [Epub ahead of print].

22. Gibson MK, Li Y, Murphy B, et al. Randomized phase III evaluation of cisplatin plus fluorouracil versus cisplatin plus paclitaxel in advanced head and neck cancer (E1395): an Intergroup trial of the Eastern Cooperative Oncology Group. J Clin Oncol 2005;23:3562–7.

23. Jacobs C, Lyman G, Velez-Garcia E, et al. A phase III randomized study comparing cisplatin and fluorouracil as single agents and in combination for advanced squamous cell carcinoma of the head and neck. J Clin Oncol 1992; 10:257–63.

24. Malhotra B, Moon J, Kucuk O, et al. Phase II trial of biweekly gemcitabine and paclitaxel with recurrent or metastatic squamous cell carcinoma of the head and neck. Southwest Oncology Group study S0329. Head Neck 2014;36:1712–7.

25. Hitt R, Irigoyen A, Cortes-Funes H, et al. Phase II study of the combination of cetuximab and weekly paclitaxel in the first-line treatment of patients with recurrent and/or metastatic squamous cell carcinoma of head and neck. Ann Oncol 2012; 23:1016–22.

26. Vermorken JB, Mesia R, Rivera F, et al. Platinum-based chemotherapy plus cetuximab in head and neck cancer. N Engl J Med 2008;359:1116–27.

27. Vermorken JB, Stohlmacher-Williams J, Davidenko I, et al. Cisplatin and fluoro-uracil with or without panitumumab in patients with recurrent or metastatic squamous-cell carcinoma of the head and neck (SPECTRUM): an open-label phase 3 randomised trial. Lancet Oncol 2013;14:697–710.

28. Ferris RL, Blumenschein G Jr, Fayette J, et al. Nivolumab for recurrent squamous-cell carcinoma of the head and neck. N Engl J Med 2016;375:1856–67.

29. US Food and Drug Administration (FDA). DA approval statement for pembrolizu-mab (Keytruda). Available at: https://www.fda.gov/drugs/informationondrugs/approveddrugs/ucm515627.htm. Accessed April 13, 2017.

30. Mehra R, Seiwert TY, Mahipal A, et al. Efficacy and safety of pembrolizumab in recurrent/metastatic head and neck squamous cell carcinoma (R/M HNSCC): pooled analyses after long-term follow-up in KEYNOTE-012. J Clin Oncol 2016; 34(Suppl 15); abstr 6012.

31. Vermorken JB, Trigo J, Hitt R, et al. Open-label, uncontrolled, multicenter phase II study to evaluate the efficacy and toxicity of cetuximab as a single agent in pa-tients with recurrent and/or metastatic squamous cell carcinoma of the head and neck who failed to respond to platinum-based therapy. J Clin Oncol 2007;25: 2171–7.

32. Cohen EE, Kane MA, List MA, et al. Phase II trial of gefitinib 250mg daily in pa-tients with recurrent and/or metastatic squamous cell carcinoma of the head and neck. Clin Cancer Res 2005;11:8418–24.

33. Stewart JS, Cohen EE, Licitra L, et al. Phase III study of gefitinib compared with intravenous methotrexate for recurrent squamous cell carcinoma of the head and neck [corrected]. J Clin Oncol 2009;27:1864–71.

34. Machiels JP, Haddad RI, Fayette J, et al. Afatinib versus methotrexate as second-line treatment in patients with recurrent or metastatic squamous-cell carcinoma of the head and neck progressing on or after platinum-based therapy (LUX-Head&-Neck 1): an open-label, randomised phase 3 trial. Lancet Oncol 2015;16:583–94.

35. Machiels JP, Henry S, Zanetta S, et al. Phase II study of sunitinib in recurrent or metastatic squamous cell carcinoma of the head and neck: GORTEC 2006-01. J Clin Oncol 2010;28:21–8.

36. Soulieres D, Senzer NN, Vokes EE, et al. Multicenter phase II study of erlotinib, an oral epidermal growth factor receptor tyrosine kinase inhibitor, in patients with recurrent or metastatic squamous cell carcinoma of the head and neck. J Clin Oncol 2004;22:77–85.

37. Catimel G, Vermorken JB, Clavel M, et al. A phase II study of Gemcitabine (LY 188011) in patients with advanced squamous cell carcinoma of the head and neck. EORTC Early Clinical Trials Group. Ann Oncol 1994;5:543–7.

38. Grau JJ, Caballero M, Verger E, et al. Weekly paclitaxel for platin-resistant stage IV head and neck cancer patients. Acta Otolaryngol 2009;129:1294–9.

39. Guardiola E, Peyrade F, Chaigneau L, et al. Results of a randomised phase II study comparing docetaxel with methotrexate in patients with recurrent head and neck cancer. Eur J Cancer 2004;40:2071–6.

Radiation Therapy for Oral Cavity and Oropharyngeal Cancers

Alexander Lin, MD

KEYWORDS

- Oral cavity cancer • Oropharyngeal cancer • Head and neck cancer
- Radiation therapy • Intensity-modulated radiation therapy

KEY POINTS

- Radiotherapy is a common modality used in the treatment of oral cavity and oropharyngeal cancers.
- The side effects of radiation, during and after treatment, can be significant and can negatively impact patient function and quality of life.
- Efforts to improve outcomes, such as through patient education, supportive care, and posttreatment adherence to rehabilitative and preventive care, can help mitigate toxicity and improve outcomes.
- Advances in radiation delivery, such as through continued technological advances, or novel approaches to customizing radiation dose and volume, to maximize the therapeutic efficacy while minimizing side effects, are warranted.

INTRODUCTION

Cancers of the oral cavity and the oropharynx exemplify the changing demographics, biology, and causes of head and neck cancer. Although cancers of the oral cavity remain largely tobacco induced, the incidence of this diagnosis continues to decrease. In contrast, the incidence of oropharyngeal cancer has been steadily increasing, largely caused by human papillomavirus (HPV) infection. Long-term disease outcomes are increasingly divergent, reflecting the different biology from HPV-associated and nonassociated tumors. This article summarizes current approaches to radiotherapy (RT) management of oral cavity and oropharyngeal cancer and highlights future efforts.

Disclosure: The author has nothing to disclose.
Department of Radiation Oncology, Perelman School of Medicine, University of Pennsylvania, 3400 Civic Center Boulevard, TRC 2-West, Philadelphia, PA 19104, USA
E-mail address: alexander.lin@uphs.upenn.edu

Dent Clin N Am 62 (2018) 99–109
http://dx.doi.org/10.1016/j.cden.2017.08.007
0011-8532/18/© 2017 Elsevier Inc. All rights reserved.

dental.theclinics.com

PRERADIATION PATIENT MANAGEMENT

Before the initiation of radiation, there are several important issues that should be addressed in order to facilitate therapy and ensure optimal long-term disease- and treatment-related outcomes.

Many patients with cancers of the oral cavity have a history of previous and/or current heavy tobacco use. From a cancer therapy–specific standpoint, continuation of smoking throughout RT has been associated with worse outcomes.[1,2] Continued smoking can also negatively impact or predispose to other comorbid conditions, such as cardiovascular disease,[3] second primary cancers,[4] and chronic obstructive pulmonary disease.[5] Efforts to intervene, motivate, and educate patients on the importance of smoking cessation are, therefore, warranted.

All patients undergoing RT to the head and neck region should receive a thorough pretreatment dental evaluation to assess if any dental treatment is required before initiation of RT to minimize the potential for dental complications during or post-RT. For example, extraction of at-risk teeth is indicated before initiation of RT to minimize the risk of osteoradionecrosis associated with postradiation dental extractions.[6] Because of the radiation exposure of salivary glands during treatment, one of the most commonly reported long-term side effects of RT is xerostomia, which significantly increases the risk of dental caries.[7,8] Therefore, an additional benefit of pre-RT dental evaluation is to receive any prescribed treatment recommendations (such as supplemental, prescription fluoride) and education on preventive posttreatment dental care to minimize the long-term dental effects from RT.

The effects of RT can negatively impact long-term speech and swallowing function as well as patient quality of life. Speech difficulties can result from muscle fibrosis, co-ordination, and strength impacting speech production. Problems with dysphagia and oral intake can result from trismus and poor coordination of muscles associated with swallowing and can predispose patients to issues such as poor nutrition or aspiration. Therefore, it is important that all patients are evaluated before radiation in order to develop a customized protocol to strengthen muscle and maintain function. These protocols, when started and maintained throughout the course of radiation, have been associated with improved posttreatment swallowing outcomes.[9]

ORAL CAVITY CANCER

Cancers of the oral cavity are commonly associated with tobacco use or may be due to local irritants (such as betel nut chewing) and, unlike oropharyngeal cancers, are usually pathologically HPV negative.[10] The estimated incidence of oral cavity cancers in the United States for 2017 is 32,670, with an estimated 6695 deaths,[11] with the incidence of HPV-negative head and neck cancers decreasing over the past several decades,[12] mirroring the decreased incidence of smoking in the population.[4] Surgery is typically the treatment of choice, as it is generally associated with improved survival compared with a definitive, nonsurgical approach.[13] Definitive RT is generally reserved for patients who are unable to undergo surgery. RT is indicated in the postoperative setting (for locally advanced-stage disease or for adverse pathologic risk factors), with or without chemotherapy, to improve disease control.

Definitive Radiotherapy for Oral Cavity Cancer

Although initial surgery is the preferred initial treatment of choice, there will be patients for whom surgical resection is not feasible (due to surgically unresectable tumor and/or medical comorbidities). For these patients, RT is a viable, definitive treatment option for oral cavity cancer. For patients receiving definitive chemoradiation (CRT) for locally advanced disease, acceptable disease outcomes and overall function were obtained for most patients[14,15] and similar to those receiving surgery.[14] For patients receiving RT alone, altered fractionations schemes (whereby the daily or total dose of radiation or total number of radiation treatment fractions are altered vs the standard dose of 1 treatment of 2 Gy daily for 35 fractions) are superior to standard fractionation. The phase III randomized study (Radiation Therapy Oncology Group [RTOG] 9003) of 4 fractionation regimens of RT alone for locally advanced, squamous cell carcinoma of the head and neck demonstrated that hyperfractionation (1.2 Gy per fraction, twice a day, 5 days a week to 81.6 Gy per 68 fractions for 7 weeks) yielded the best long-term results with respect to locoregional control and overall survival.[16] The DAHANCA 6 and 7 studies, a comparison of 6 versus 5 weekly treatments, demonstrated that 6 treatments weekly yielded superior 5-year locoregional control (70% vs 60%) and disease-specific survival (73% vs 66%).[17]

Postoperative External Beam Radiotherapy for Oral Cavity Cancer

The indications for requiring postoperative RT for oral cavity cancer include pathologic factors, such as (1) margin status, (2) the presence of perineural of lympho-vascular invasion, and (3) overall cancer stage. For those with these factors, postoperative RT is considered the standard of care and has been shown to reduce the rates of disease recurrence and improve survival.[18] Two large multicenter randomized trials (European Organization for Research and Treatment of Cancer [EORTC] 22931 and RTOG 9501) demonstrated the importance of postoperative RT after resection of advanced-stage disease (stages III–IV), showing improved overall survival (EORTC 22931)[19] and locoregional control (RTOG 9501)[20] with the addition of postoperative RT. In the presence of nodal extracapsular extension and/or positive surgical margins, the addition of concurrent cisplatin-based chemotherapy improves locoregional control and overall survival versus RT alone.[21]

Evidence Basis for Safety/Toxicity

Long-term results of RTOG 9003 showed that, in the most efficacious arm (hyperfractionation) with respect to disease control, there was a less than 10% grade 3 to 5 toxicity at 5 years, with less than 5% feeding tube dependency.[16] Single-institution series provide more information about late toxicities with intensity-modulated RT (IMRT), which demonstrates favorable safety/toxicity profiles.

- Of the 42 patients treated with IMRT at the Dana-Farber Cancer Institute (30 treated with surgical followed by postoperative radiation, 12 treated definitively with RT ± chemotherapy), the following grade 3 or greater acute toxicities were observed: 93% mucositis, 10% dermatitis, 83% esophagitis, 5% soft tissue. Severe (≥grade 3) late toxicities were uncommon: 19% dysphagia, 0% xerostomia, and 2% bone and soft tissue damage.[15]
- Results from the Memorial Sloan-Kettering Cancer of postoperative oral cavity IMRT (median dose 60 Gy) showed the following rates of grade 3 or greater acute toxicities[22]: 3% dermatitis, 23% mucositis, 0% xerostomia, 6% esophagitis. The following rates of grade 3 or greater late toxicities were reported: 0% mandible or larynx damage, trismus, 6% xerostomia.[22]

The acute toxicities of RT for oral cavity cancer are generally reported in the categories of mucositis, pharyngitis, dysphagia, odynophagia, and xerostomia. These side effects are common during a standard course of radiation and rarely life-threatening. A late effect of particular concern for radiation to the oral cavity is osteoradionecrosis, given the close proximity of the mandible to the primary tumor site.

Older series report a 14% to 18% rate of osteonecrosis, but recent series using IMRT report much lower rates of 0% to 2%[15,22]

Treatment with IMRT has shown an excellent toxicity profile, reflecting the finding that the survival rate of oral cavity cancers has improved over the past 2 decades, presumably because of technological advances in therapy.[23]

OROPHARYNGEAL CANCER

Cancers of the oropharynx were traditionally associated with tobacco use but are now increasingly due to exposure to and infection with HPV. The incidence of HPV-associated oropharyngeal cancers has been increasing over the past several decades, with middle-aged men comprising most of the diagnoses.[12] Most of these patients report little or no history of tobacco use; long-term outcomes after treatment, even with advanced-stage disease, is outstanding, with most of the patients cured.[24,25] The new staging system for oropharyngeal cancer will soon reflect these differences in outcomes due to HPV, with staging reflecting the presence or absence of HPV.[26]

For early stage lesions of the oropharynx, treatment with RT has provided excellent rates of local control. Many patients will receive treatment with RT in place of surgery, depending on the expected functional outcome associated with surgical resection. For patients with advanced-stage disease, RT can be used as the definitive treatment modality (often with concurrent chemotherapy), or as adjuvant therapy after initial surgical resection.

Radiotherapy Alone for Early Stage Disease

Large single-institution series have demonstrated high rates of locoregional control with RT alone for oropharyngeal cancer, particularly those with early stage disease. In the pre-IMRT era, local control rates of 94% for T1 disease and 79% for T2 disease were obtained,[27] whereas results from a more modern RT era yielded 5-year local control rates of 82% for T1 disease and 74% for T2 disease, which compare favorably with primary surgical series.[28]

RTOG 00-22, a multi-institutional trial of accelerated hypofractionated IMRT (without chemotherapy) for early stage oropharyngeal cancer demonstrated that moderately accelerated hypofractionated IMRT was feasible, with high disease control rates (locoregional failure rates of <10%) and reduced salivary toxicity compared with similar patients treated in previous RTOG studies.[29]

Definitive Radiotherapy Alone for Locally Advanced Disease

Similar to the benefits described earlier for patients with oral cavity cancer, in patients with advanced-stage oropharyngeal cancer receiving RT alone, altered fractionation schemes are superior to standard fractionation. A meta-analysis of standard versus altered fractionation RT showed that 5-year survival was improved with altered fractionation RT (3.4%), suggesting the greatest benefit with hyperfractionation (8% at 5 years).[30]

Definitive Chemoradiation for Locally Advanced Disease

Several trials[31,32] and a meta-analysis[33] have compared CRT with radiation alone or concurrent cetuximab with radiation versus radiation alone[34,35] for organ-preservation therapy of locally advanced oropharyngeal cancer. These studies demonstrated superiority of CRT over RT alone (6% overall survival benefit at 5 years in the randomized trials, 8% overall survival benefit of CRT over RT alone in the meta-analysis) as well as cetuximab/RT over RT alone (9% survival benefit at 5 years). For patients who are to receive an organ-preservation treatment approach, current standards of care suggest that concurrent chemotherapy (platinum based) should be given with RT as the first-line treatment, reserving cetuximab for those who cannot tolerate standard chemotherapy, and RT alone for those who cannot tolerate or refuse both standard chemotherapy and cetuximab.

Postoperative External Beam Radiotherapy for Oropharyngeal Cancer

In the setting of a resected, locally advanced oropharyngeal cancer, postoperative EBRT reduces the rates of disease recurrence and improves survival.[18] Two large multicenter randomized trials (EORTC 22931 and RTOG 9501) demonstrated the importance of postoperative RT after resection of advanced-stage disease (stages III–IV), showing improved overall survival (EORTC 22931)[19] and locoregional control (RTOG 9501)[20] with the addition of postoperative RT. In the presence of nodal extracapsular extension and/ or positive surgical margins, the addition of concurrent cisplatin-based chemotherapy improves locoregional control and overall survival versus RT alone.[21]

Intensity-Modulated Radiation Therapy

IMRT is a method of radiation delivery in which multiple individual radiation beamlets are optimized in intensity to provide the best possible radiation plan in terms of treatment areas of cancer, while minimizing exposure of adjacent critical normal organs and tissues (**Fig. 1**). IMRT is now commonly used in the treatment of oropharyngeal cancer, given the excellent local control outcomes and normal tissue-sparing capabilities. One of the largest single-institution reports of IMRT for stages III and IV oropharyngeal cancer from the University of California-San Francisco demonstrated a 3-year locoregional control rate of 90%.[36] GORTEC 2004-03, a multicenter prospective study of IMRT in head and neck cancer, on which 117 patients with oropharyngeal cancer were treated with IMRT, reported a 2-year locoregional control rate of 86%.[37] Furthermore, studies have shown that IMRT can be delivered safely and effectively outside of a specialized academic setting, demonstrating its general applicability.[38] The results of these studies are consistent with the overall excellent prognosis and low rates of locoregional failure observed in patients with oropharyngeal cancer (particularly those with

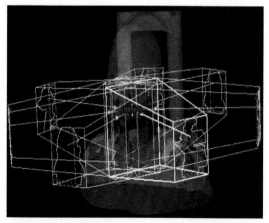

Fig. 1. Patient with a stage IVa oropharynx cancer. IMRT for definitive RT to the primary site and bilateral neck, using 7 coplanar, equidistant beams with multi-leaf collimator.

HPV-induced disease) treated in large randomized trials, such as the RTOG 0129,[24] or in large institutional series, such as the one from the Princess Margaret Hospital.[25]

Evidence Basis for Safety/Toxicity

The recent literature on treatment results with IMRT is the most accurate gauge of safety/toxicity with currently used techniques and technology for oropharyngeal cancer RT.

- In the University of California-San Francisco series, acute grade 3 or 4 toxicities were observed in 35 (49.0%) patients, with only 1 (1.4%) patient experiencing a grade 3 or 4 late toxicity.[36]
- In the GORTEC 2004-03 study, feeding tube dependency at 12 months was 4% and 2% experienced osteoradionecrosis.[37]
- The University of Michigan series of 73 patients with stage III or IV oropharyngeal cancer treated with IMRT (used to spare dose to swallowing structures) and concurrent chemotherapy at the University of Michigan reported that at 1 year after therapy, observer-rated dysphagia was absent or minimal in all but 4 (5.5%) patients.[39]

Randomized controlled trials have compared IMRT with non-IMRT techniques and have consistently demonstrated superiority of IMRT with respect to improved long-term xerostomia[40,41] and global quality of life.[40] Furthermore, multi-institutional data of more than 2300 patients treated demonstrate that modern nonsurgical treatment of oropharyngeal cancer is associated with a very low rate (3.7% at 2 years) of long-term feeding tube dependence.[42]

Recent advances in technology can potentially improve the safety profile of IMRT. For example, the use of volumetric modulated arc therapy for IMRT, when compared with fixed field IMRT, can improve conformity of dose targeted areas, while improving sparing of salivary gland structures and reducing patient exposure by decreasing the amount of delivered monitor units of radiation.[43]

Future Directions

Although IMRT is a well-established and commonly utilized modality in the treatment of oropharyngeal cancer, conventional RT is associated with acute and late toxicity, with critical normal organs and tissues receiving significant radiation exposure because of the close proximity of disease. Significant late effects of RT,[44–50] although not common, can cause significant morbidity and impact posttreatment quality of life.[46] In an era when the epidemiology of oropharyngeal cancer is changing, with an increasing proportion of younger patients developing HPV-positive oropharyngeal cancer treated with excellent long-term disease outcomes,[24,25] minimizing long-term treatment-related complications is increasingly important.

Approaches to improving the therapeutic ratio of treatment, minimizing toxicity while maintaining high rates of cancer control, are the subject of multiple current clinical studies for oropharyngeal cancer, investigating alternative approaches for each treatment modality (surgery, chemotherapy, and RT).

Current investigations and methods to diminishing toxicity include (1) substitution of alternative agent chemotherapy or omitting chemotherapy altogether, (2) reducing the volume of tissue electively radiated, (3) reducing the dose of radiation prescribed, or (4) applying new/emerging technologies in radiation delivery. The RTOG 1016 (closed to accrual, final results pending) is investigating whether substituting cetuximab for cisplatin in patients receiving organ-preservation RT yields equivalent disease outcomes with less toxicity.[51] The NRG HN002 study for definitive RT is using 60 Gy

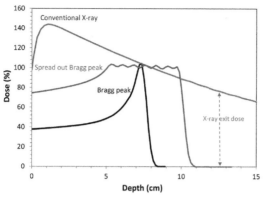

Fig. 2. Comparison of depth dose profiles of a conventional radiation x-ray beam (*orange*), a monoenergetic proton beam (*black*), and a poly-energetic proton beam with a spread-out Bragg peak (*blue*).

for all patients, allows for ipsilateral neck RT for selected patients with well-lateralized tonsil cancers, and is investigating whether RT alone is equivalent to RT + cisplatin.[52] Postoperatively, studies are examining both the possible role of volume reduction (actively omitting high-dose RT to the resected primary tumor bed in well-selected patients with small, completely resected primary oropharyngeal tumors, while delivering full-dose RT to the nodal regions in the neck[53]) or decreasing the dose of RT from the standard dose of 60 Gy to 50 Gy (ECOG 3311).[54] Finally, new technologies, such as proton RT, can be used in conjunction with other approaches to further improve normal tissue sparing from high-dose radiation. This sparing is due to the unique physical nature of proton therapy limiting the area of high-dose radiation, resulting in less dose delivered to tissues proximal to the tumor and rapid dose falloff at the distal edge of the tumor (Bragg-Peak effect, **Fig. 2**). This dose falloff allows for potential significant sparing of critical structures (such as the salivary glands, swallowing musculature, mandible, oral cavity) that when overexposed, can lead to severe acute (odynophagia, mucositis) and long-term side effects (dysphagia, xerostomia, dysgeusia) associated with conventional RT techniques (**Fig. 3**). Although promising, the full clinical benefits

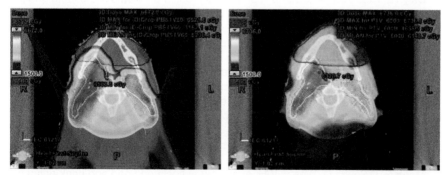

Fig. 3. A 58-year-old man with a diagnosis of a pathologic stage IVa, T2N2bM0, HPV-positive squamous cell carcinoma of the right tonsil. Postoperative proton radiation therapy was delivered using a 2-beam posterior-oblique approach (*shown on the left*), with the comparative IMRT plan shown on the right. Dose color was set to lower threshold of 15 Gy. The mean dose delivered to oral cavity (*purple*) with proton therapy was 3 Gy. The IMRT plan would have delivered a mean dose of 19 Gy to the oral cavity.

associated with technological advances, such as proton therapy, will be best characterized by current and future efforts using comparative outcomes and/or prospective trials comparing proton therapy versus the most advanced, photon-based RT delivery methods.

SUMMARY

RT is a well-established and often-used therapeutic modality for the treatment of oral cavity and oropharyngeal cancers. When used in the postoperative setting, it has demonstrated benefits in improving disease control and survival. When used in place of surgery, it has demonstrated that it is an effective alternative to surgery without compromising disease outcomes; however, the effects of therapy on patient function and quality of life remains an issue. Integration of pre-RT patient education and rehabilitative and preventative care should be considered standard and can help facilitate a quicker and more complete recovery. Novel radiotherapeutic investigations, such as new technologies, as well as customization of radiation dose and volume, are of importance moving forward if we are to continue to improve outcomes.

REFERENCES

1. Browman GP, Wong G, Hodson I, et al. Influence of cigarette smoking on the efficacy of radiation therapy in head and neck cancer. N Engl J Med 1993;328: 159–63.
2. Gillison ML, Zhang Q, Jordan R, et al. Tobacco smoking and increased risk of death and progression for patients with p16-positive and p16-negative oropharyngeal cancer. J Clin Oncol 2012;30:2102–11.
3. Jee SH, Suh I, Kim IS, et al. Smoking and atherosclerotic cardiovascular disease in men with low levels of serum cholesterol: the Korea Medical Insurance Corporation Study. JAMA 1999;282:2149–55.
4. Alberg AJ, Samet JM. Epidemiology of lung cancer. Chest 2003;123:21S–49S.
5. Lokke A, Lange P, Scharling H, et al. Developing COPD: a 25 year follow up study of the general population. Thorax 2006;61:935–9.
6. Thariat J, De Mones E, Darcourt V, et al. Teeth and irradiation in head and neck cancer. Cancer Radiother 2010;14:128–36 [in French].
7. Daly TE, Drane JB, MacComb WS. Management of problems of the teeth and jaw in patients undergoing irradiation. Am J Surg 1972;124:539–42.
8. Horiot JC, Schraub S, Bone MC, et al. Dental preservation in patients irradiated for head and neck tumours: a 10-year experience with topical fluoride and a randomized trial between two fluoridation methods. Radiother Oncol 1983;1:77–82.
9. Carroll WR, Locher JL, Canon CL, et al. Pretreatment swallowing exercises improve swallow function after chemoradiation. Laryngoscope 2008;118:39–43.
10. Castellsague X, Alemany L, Quer M, et al. HPV involvement in head and neck cancers: comprehensive assessment of biomarkers in 3680 patients. J Natl Cancer Inst 2016;108:djv403.
11. Siegel RL, Miller KD, Jemal A. Cancer statistics, 2017. CA Cancer J Clin 2017;67: 7–30.
12. Marur S, D'Souza G, Westra WH, et al. HPV-associated head and neck cancer: a virus-related cancer epidemic. Lancet Oncol 2010;11:781–9.
13. Iyer NG, Tan DS, Tan VK, et al. Randomized trial comparing surgery and adjuvant radiotherapy versus concurrent chemoradiotherapy in patients with advanced, nonmetastatic squamous cell carcinoma of the head and neck: 10-year update and subset analysis. Cancer 2015;121:1599–607.

14. Stenson KM, Kunnavakkam R, Cohen EE, et al. Chemoradiation for patients with advanced oral cavity cancer. Laryngoscope 2010;120:93–9.

15. Sher DJ, Thotakura V, Balboni TA, et al. Treatment of oral cavity squamous cell carcinoma with adjuvant or definitive intensity-modulated radiation therapy. Int J Radiat Oncol Biol Phys 2011;81:e215–22.

16. Beitler JJ, Zhang Q, Fu KK, et al. Final results of local-regional control and late toxicity of RTOG 9003: a randomized trial of altered fractionation radiation for locally advanced head and neck cancer. Int J Radiat Oncol Biol Phys 2014;89: 13–20.

17. Overgaard J, Hansen HS, Specht L, et al. Five compared with six fractions per week of conventional radiotherapy of squamous-cell carcinoma of head and neck: DAHANCA 6 and 7 randomised controlled trial. Lancet 2003;362:933–40.

18. Lundahl RE, Foote RL, Bonner JA, et al. Combined neck dissection and postoperative radiation therapy in the management of the high-risk neck: a matched-pair analysis. Int J Radiat Oncol Biol Phys 1998;40:529–34.

19. Bernier J, Domenge C, Ozsahin M, et al. Postoperative irradiation with or without concomitant chemotherapy for locally advanced head and neck cancer. N Engl J Med 2004;350:1945–52.

20. Cooper JS, Pajak TF, Forastiere AA, et al. Postoperative concurrent radiotherapy and chemotherapy for high-risk squamous-cell carcinoma of the head and neck. N Engl J Med 2004;350:1937–44.

21. Bernier J, Cooper JS, Pajak TF, et al. Defining risk levels in locally advanced head and neck cancers: a comparative analysis of concurrent postoperative radiation plus chemotherapy trials of the EORTC (#22931) and RTOG (# 9501). Head Neck 2005;27:843–50.

22. Gomez DR, Zhung JE, Gomez J, et al. Intensity-modulated radiotherapy in postoperative treatment of oral cavity cancers. Int J Radiat Oncol Biol Phys 2009;73: 1096–103.

23. Amit M, Yen TC, Liao CT, et al. Improvement in survival of patients with oral cavity squamous cell carcinoma: an international collaborative study. Cancer 2013;119: 4242–8.

24. Ang KK, Harris J, Wheeler R, et al. Human papillomavirus and survival of patients with oropharyngeal cancer. N Engl J Med 2010;363:24–35.

25. O'Sullivan B, Huang SH, Siu LL, et al. Deintensification candidate subgroups in human papillomavirus-related oropharyngeal cancer according to minimal risk of distant metastasis. J Clin Oncol 2013;31:543–50.

26. O'Sullivan B, Huang SH, Su J, et al. Development and validation of a staging system for HPV-related oropharyngeal cancer by the International Collaboration on Oropharyngeal Cancer Network for Staging (ICON-S): a multicentre cohort study. Lancet Oncol 2016;17:440–51.

27. Jackson SM, Hay JH, Flores AD, et al. Cancer of the tonsil: the results of ipsilateral radiation treatment. Radiother Oncol 1999;51:123–8.

28. Charbonneau N, Gelinas M, del Vecchio P, et al. Primary radiotherapy for tonsillar carcinoma: a good alternative to a surgical approach. J Otolaryngol 2006;35: 227–34.

29. Eisbruch A, Harris J, Garden AS, et al. Multi-institutional trial of accelerated hypofractionated intensity-modulated radiation therapy for early-stage oropharyngeal cancer (RTOG 00-22). Int J Radiat Oncol Biol Phys 2010;76:1333–8.

30. Bourhis J, Overgaard J, Audry H, et al. Hyperfractionated or accelerated radiotherapy in head and neck cancer: a meta-analysis. Lancet 2006;368:843–54.

31. Calais G, Alfonsi M, Bardet E, et al. Randomized trial of radiation therapy versus concomitant chemotherapy and radiation therapy for advanced-stage oropharynx carcinoma. J Natl Cancer Inst 1999;91:2081–6.
32. Denis F, Garaud P, Bardet E, et al. Final results of the 94-01 French Head and Neck Oncology and Radiotherapy Group randomized trial comparing radiotherapy alone with concomitant radiochemotherapy in advanced-stage oropharynx carcinoma. J Clin Oncol 2004;22:69–76.
33. Blanchard P, Baujat B, Holostenco V, et al. Meta-analysis of chemotherapy in head and neck cancer (MACH-NC): a comprehensive analysis by tumour site. Radiother Oncol 2011;100:33–40.
34. Bonner JA, Harari PM, Giralt J, et al. Radiotherapy plus cetuximab for squamous-cell carcinoma of the head and neck. N Engl J Med 2006;354:567–78.
35. Bonner JA, Harari PM, Giralt J, et al. Radiotherapy plus cetuximab for locoregionally advanced head and neck cancer: 5-year survival data from a phase 3 randomised trial, and relation between cetuximab-induced rash and survival. Lancet Oncol 2010;11:21–8.
36. Huang K, Xia P, Chuang C, et al. Intensity-modulated chemoradiation for treatment of stage III and IV oropharyngeal carcinoma: the University of California-San Francisco experience. Cancer 2008;113:497–507.
37. Toledano I, Graff P, Serre A, et al. Intensity-modulated radiotherapy in head and neck cancer: results of the prospective study GORTEC 2004-03. Radiother Oncol 2012;103:57–62.
38. Seung S, Bae J, Solhjem M, et al. Intensity-modulated radiotherapy for head-and-neck cancer in the community setting. Int J Radiat Oncol Biol Phys 2008;72: 1075–81.
39. Feng FY, Kim HM, Lyden TH, et al. Intensity-modulated chemoradiotherapy aiming to reduce dysphagia in patients with oropharyngeal cancer: clinical and functional results. J Clin Oncol 2010;28:2732–8.
40. Nutting CM, Morden JP, Harrington KJ, et al. Parotid-sparing intensity modulated versus conventional radiotherapy in head and neck cancer (PARSPORT): a phase 3 multicentre randomised controlled trial. Lancet Oncol 2011;12:127–36.
41. Gupta T, Agarwal J, Jain S, et al. Three-dimensional conformal radiotherapy (3D-CRT) versus intensity modulated radiation therapy (IMRT) in squamous cell carcinoma of the head and neck: a randomized controlled trial. Radiother Oncol 2012;104:343–8.
42. Setton J, Lee NY, Riaz N, et al. A multi-institution pooled analysis of gastrostomy tube dependence in patients with oropharyngeal cancer treated with definitive intensity-modulated radiotherapy. Cancer 2015;121:294–301.
43. Teoh M, Beveridge S, Wood K, et al. Volumetric-modulated arc therapy (RapidArc) vs. conventional fixed-field intensity-modulated radiotherapy for (1)(8)F-FDG-PET-guided dose escalation in oropharyngeal cancer: a planning study. Med Dosim 2013;38:18–24.
44. Dorresteijn LD, Kappelle AC, Boogerd W, et al. Increased risk of ischemic stroke after radiotherapy on the neck in patients younger than 60 years. J Clin Oncol 2002;20:282–8.
45. Eisbruch A, Lyden T, Bradford CR, et al. Objective assessment of swallowing dysfunction and aspiration after radiation concurrent with chemotherapy for head-and-neck cancer. Int J Radiat Oncol Biol Phys 2002;53:23–8.
46. Lin A, Kim HM, Terrell JE, et al. Quality of life after parotid-sparing IMRT for head-and-neck cancer: a prospective longitudinal study. Int J Radiat Oncol Biol Phys 2003;57:61–70.

47. Smith GL, Smith BD, Buchholz TA, et al. Cerebrovascular disease risk in older head and neck cancer patients after radiotherapy. J Clin Oncol 2008;26:5119–25.

48. Smith GL, Smith BD, Garden AS, et al. Hypothyroidism in older patients with head and neck cancer after treatment with radiation: a population-based study. Head Neck 2009;31:1031–8.

49. Tsai CJ, Hofstede TM, Sturgis EM, et al. Osteoradionecrosis and radiation dose to the mandible in patients with oropharyngeal cancer. Int J Radiat Oncol Biol Phys 2013;85:415–20.

50. Swisher-McClure S, Mitra N, Lin A, et al. Risk of fatal cerebrovascular accidents after external beam radiation therapy for early-stage glottic laryngeal cancer. Head Neck 2014;36:611–6.

51. Radiation Therapy Oncology Group, National Cancer Institute, NRG Oncology. Radiation therapy with cisplatin or cetuximab in treating patients with oropharyngeal cancer. Available at: https://clinicaltrials.gov/ct2/show/NCT01302834. (ClinicalTrials.gov Identifier: NCT01302834). Accessed June 23, 2017.

52. NRG Oncology, National Cancer Institute. Reduced-dose intensity-modulated radiation therapy with or without cisplatin in treating patients with advanced oropharyngeal cancer. Available at: https://clinicaltrials.gov/ct2/show/NCT02254278 (ClinicalTrials. gov Identifier: NCT02254278). Accessed June 23, 2017.

53. Abramson Cancer Center, University of Pennsylvania. A single-arm phase II study of post-transoral robotic surgery (TORS) alone to the primary tumor site and selective neck dissection (SND) followed by adjuvant radiation therapy (±Chemotherapy) to the regional nodes for advanced stage, human papilloma virus (HPV) positive, oropharyngeal cancer. Available at: https://clinicaltrials. gov/ct2/show/NCT02159703. (ClinicalTrials.gov Identifier: NCT02159703). Accessed June 23, 2017.

54. Eastern Cooperative Oncology Group, National Cancer Institute. Transoral surgery followed by low-dose or standard-dose radiation therapy with or without chemotherapy in treating patients with HPV positive stage III-IVA oropharyngeal cancer. Available at: https://clinicaltrials.gov/ct2/show/NCT01898494 (ClinicalTrials.gov Identifier: NCT01898494). Accessed June 23, 2017.

Human Papillomavirus and Oropharyngeal Cancer

Takako Imai Tanaka, DDS, FDS RCSEd[a],*, Faizan Alawi, DDS[b]

KEYWORDS

- Human papillomavirus • Oropharyngeal cancer • Oral squamous cell carcinoma
- Tonsillar cancer • HPV 16 • p16

KEY POINTS

- Human papillomavirus (HPV) infection is a distinct risk factor for oropharyngeal squamous cell carcinoma (OPSCC), and HPV 16 is associated with most HPV-OPSCC cases.
- Incidence rate of HPV-OPSCC, particularly tonsillar cancer, has been rapidly increasing for the past 2 decades, whereas tobacco-related head and neck squamous cell carcinoma rates are decreasing worldwide.
- Typical patients with HPV-OPSCC are described as men, white, younger than 60, healthier individuals with no or little tobacco exposure, and having a higher socioeconomic status.
- Strong association between orogenital contact and OPSCC was found in a hospital-based, case-control study. A recent systematic review in 2014 found 50% to 80% of adolescents and young adults reported participation in oral sex.
- The potential benefit of HPV vaccination to reduce the risk of HPV-OPSCC has been suggested.

INTRODUCTION

The link between human papillomavirus (HPV) infection and head and neck squamous cell carcinoma (HNSCC) was first described by Syrjanen and colleagues[1] in 1983. However, in some of the historic HPV literature, distinctions were not made between cancers arising in the oral cavity and oropharynx. It is now well established that HPV infection is a significant risk factor for the development of oropharyngeal squamous cell carcinoma (OPSCC); furthermore, HPV-associated OPSCC (HPV-OPSCC) is recognized as a unique subtype of HNSCC comprising approximately 25% of all

Disclosure Statement: The authors have no commercial or financial conflicts of interest and no funding sources to disclose.
[a] Department of Oral Medicine, University of Pennsylvania School of Dental Medicine, 240 South 40th Street, Robert Schattner Center #215, Philadelphia, PA 19104, USA; [b] Department of Pathology, University of Pennsylvania School of Dental Medicine, 240 South 40th Street, 328B, Philadelphia, PA 19104, USA
* Corresponding author.
E-mail address: takakot@upenn.edu

HNSCC.[2] Epidemiologic studies have shown increasing incidence rates of HPV-OPSCC for the last 2 decades, whereas tobacco-related HNSCC rates are decreasing worldwide.[3–5] In the near future, the global burden of HPV-OPSCC is predicted to surpass that of cervical cancer, in which HPV infection is also known to be etiologic.[6]

It is estimated that approximately 70% of all OPSCC are linked to HPV infection.[7] In contrast, HPV is not considered to be a major risk factor for the development of *oral cavity* squamous cell carcinoma (OSCC). A meta-analysis (from a total of 4680 samples from 94 studies) reported the probability of detecting HPV in benign leukoplakia as 22% and in dysplastic lesions as 26.2%.[8] However, studies suggest that HPV contributes to the pathogenesis of only a very small subset (1%–10%) of all OSCC.[4,9,10] Tobacco and alcohol remain the major risk factors for OSCC. The important distinctions between OPSCC and OSCC are now reflected in the recently published 4th edition of the World Health Organization (WHO) Classification of Tumours of the Head and Neck[11] as well as in the 8th edition of the American Joint Committee on Cancer (AJCC) Staging Manual.[12] The clinical staging criteria for HPV-OPSCC have been significantly revised to accommodate current understanding of these cancers. The changes reflect the uniqueness of HPV-OPSCC, including site specificity, demographics, clinical features, and response to treatment when compared with non–HPV-OPSCC. This review describes current understanding of the link between HPV infection and OPSCC, with updated biological and clinical evidence.

HUMAN PAPILLOMAVIRUS–ASSOCIATED HEAD AND NECK SQUAMOUS CELL CARCINOMA: EPIDEMIOLOGY AND CLINICAL CHARACTERISTICS

HPV is a small (8-kb), nonenveloped circular DNA virus with epithelial tropism.[13] The HPV family comprises approximately 200 viral strains with more than 40 being transmitted through direct contact with the skin and mucous membranes.[13,14] To this end, HPV infection is the most common sexually transmitted disease in the United States. According to the Centers for Disease Control and Prevention (CDC), approximately 20 million Americans are currently infected with HPV with 6 million newly infected each year.[7] Nearly all sexually active individuals will acquire an HPV infection at some point in their lives.[3] Although most HPV infections are typically cleared by the host's immune system within 1 to 2 years without causing any symptoms, some persist for months to years.[15]

Depending on its ability to persist and transform infected epithelial cells, HPV is divided into 2 broad subtypes: high-risk and low-risk HPV.[15] Low-risk HPV, including HPV 6 and 11, is associated with benign lesions such as verruca vulgaris or condyloma acuminatum (**Fig. 1**). High-risk HPV is associated with malignancy, mostly in the cervix, vulva, vagina, penis, anus, rectum, and oropharynx, including the base of tongue and tonsil.[16] The WHO currently identifies 12 HPV strains (types 16, 18, 31, 33, 35, 39, 45, 51, 52, 56, 58, and 59) as high-risk cancer-causing types.[15]

HPV types 16 and 18 are associated with the vast majority of HPV-related cancers in the United States; HPV 16 is now recognized as a carcinogenic agent for OPSCC.[16–19] In contrast, HPV types 31, 33, 45, 52, and 58, combined, are linked to approximately 10% of all HPV-positive cancers.[17] A recent CDC study reported that almost 39,000 HPV-associated cancers (11.7 per 100,000 persons) were annually diagnosed during the period from 2008 to 2012; approximately 40% of these were diagnosed as OPSCC[20] (**Fig. 2**). Collectively, the incidence rates of HPV-OPSCC have been increasing for the last 3 decades, whereas tobacco-related HNSCC rates are decreasing worldwide.[3,4] The increase in incidence of OPSCC in relation to all HNSCC is significant; HPV-OPSCC increased at a rate of 2.5% per year in the United States

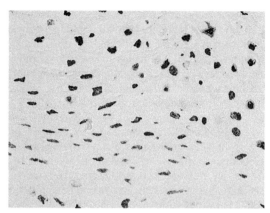

Fig. 1. Oral condyloma acuminatum exhibiting HPV-infected cells. Nuclei of the superficial keratinocytes are positive for HPV (viral strain unknown) as evaluated by immunohistochemistry (original magnification ×400).

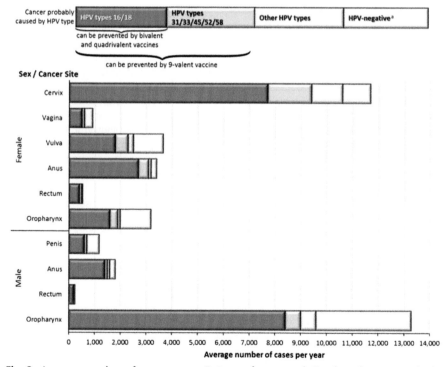

Fig. 2. Average number of cancer cases. Data are from population-based cancer registries participating in the CDC National Program of Cancer Registries or the NCI Surveillance, Epidemiology, and End Results program for all years 2009 to 2013 and cover about 99% of the US population. (*From* Centers for Disease Control and Prevention (CDC). Number of HPV-attributable cancer cases per year. Available at: https://www.cdc.gov/cancer/hpv/statistics/cases.htm. Accessed June 30, 2017.)

from 2002 to 2012.[21] Overall, there was a 26.6% increase in incidence of OPSCC from 1975 through 2012.[5] In an analysis of data from 23 countries, the increased incidence of OPSCC was predominant in economically developed counties, including the United States, Australia, Canada, Japan, and Slovakia.[22] The recent dramatic increase in the incidence of tonsillar and base of tongue cancer is also noteworthy. Its annual incidence in the United States was found to be 5% of all HNSCC,[6] and a study in Sweden showed tonsillar cancer increased its share of HNSCC from 28% to 68% during the years 1970 to 2002.[23]

Typical patients with HPV-OPSCC are described as being younger than 60, men, white and non-Hispanic, healthier individuals with no or little tobacco exposure, and having a higher socioeconomic status.[20,24] Sexual behavior, including a high number of lifetime sex partners, an increase in oral sex practices, same-sex contact, and earlier age at sexual debut, has been suggested as reasons for this trend.[25] The global burden of HPV-OPSCC is predicted to surpass the burden of cervical cancer in the near future, especially as the incident rate of HPV-OPSCC continues to increase in patients over the age of 65.[26]

HIGH-RISK HUMAN PAPILLOMAVIRUS INFECTION AND PATHOGENESIS

The likelihood of detecting high-risk HPV in OPSCC has been reported as higher than in healthy normal mucosa.[2,8,14] However, the mechanisms through which high-risk HPV infection contributes to carcinogenesis remain under active investigation. The reticulated crypt epithelium of the lingual and palatine tonsils strongly expresses programmed cell death-1 ligand 1 (PD1-L1). PD1-L1 suppresses the T-cell response to HPV, thereby creating an "immune-privileged" site for infection and adaptive immune resistance to the virus. Persistence and propagation of the virus may eventually lead to carcinogenesis.[27]

The oncogenic activity of high-risk HPV is mainly linked to expression of its viral oncoproteins E6 and E7 in the tumor cells.[18] E6 binds to p53 and targets it for degradation, whereas E7 binds and promotes degradation of retinoblastoma (pRb) tumor suppressor protein. There is a cooperative effect between the p53 and pRb molecular pathways; together they regulate essentially all critical biologic functions required for normal cellular homeostasis. A detailed discussion of p53 and pRb is beyond the scope of the current review.

The pRb signaling pathways is directly regulated by the p16 tumor suppressor protein (CDKN2A); p16 also indirectly regulates the p53 pathway (**Fig. 3**). Hyperphosphorylation of pRb causes the release of active, free E2F, which, in turn, activates several genes that control DNA synthesis. p16 binds and inhibits cyclin-dependent kinases (CDK) 4 and 6, thereby abrogating the catalytic activity of the CDK-cyclin D1 complexes that are normally required for pRb phosphorylation; this triggers cell-cycle arrest. Mutation or deletion of p16 or methylation of its promoter, which are common occurrences in neoplasia, including HNSCC, lead to loss of p16 function. This is considered biologically equivalent to loss of pRb function. Furthermore, loss of pRb function following HPV infection leads to upregulation of p16 via a feedback mechanism.

Overexpression of p16 protein as determined by immunohistochemistry is considered a reliable surrogate of HPV infection in evaluation of OPSCC tissue samples.[2,13,28] A tumor is characterized as being p16 positive if there is strong (+2/3 staining intensity) and diffuse nuclear and cytoplasmic staining of more than 70% of the malignant cells (**Fig. 4**).[12,29] This threshold and scoring system have been validated by numerous studies and in meta-analyses. A finding of only

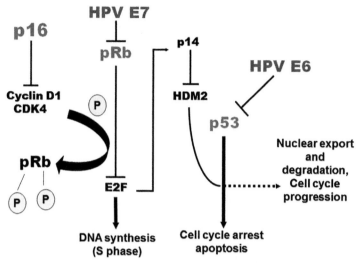

Fig. 3. HPV E6 and E7 disrupt the pRb and p53 molecular pathways. HPV E6 inactivates p53, whereas HPV E7 inactivates pRb. p16 plays an important role in upstream regulation of pRb. Loss pRb activity results in overexpression of p16. A detailed review of the proteins and pathways illustrated here are discussed in Macaluso and colleagues. (*Data from* Macaluso M, Montanari M, Cinti C, et al. Modulation of cell cycle components by epigenetic and genetic events. Semin Oncol 2005;32:452–7.)

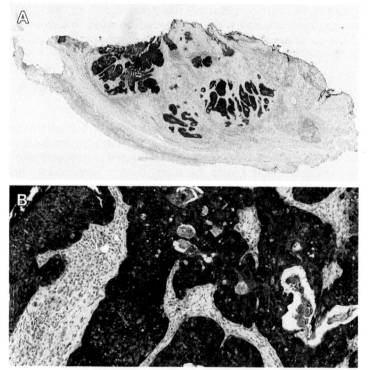

Fig. 4. Strong and diffuse cytoplasmic and nuclear p16 staining in OPSCC. (*A*) (Hematoxylin, original magnification ×20). (*B*) (Hematoxylin, original magnification ×200).

cytoplasmic p16 staining is considered to be nondiagnostic, and the tumor is described as being "negative" for HPV in this context. p16 overexpression is also considered an independent positive predictor of survival in patients with HPV-positive OPSCC.[28,30] Interestingly, p16 overexpression may also be associated with increased survival in patients with HPV-negative carcinomas of other head and neck sites, including the oral cavity.[28] Moreover, pRb can be inactivated via mechanisms other than HPV.[28,31] However, the significance of p16 overexpression in HPV-negative neoplasia requires further study before it can be applied in the clinical setting.

Although p16 expression is a surrogate of HPV infection, the gold standard remains detection of HPV E6 and E7 messenger RNA (mRNA) expression via quantitative reverse transcription polymerase chain reaction PCR (qRT-PCR); this is indicative of transcriptionally active virus within tumor cells.[18] In one study, transcriptionally active HPV was detected in 56% of OPSCC but less than 1% of OSCC.[32] Elevated levels of E6 and E7 mRNA have been found to be directly related to increasing severity of the disease in many cases of cervical cancer.[33,34] Detection of HPV DNA by in situ hybridization can also be used to assess HPV status. However, this method is not nearly as sensitive as qRT-PCR, and it reflects only the presence of viral DNA rather than transcriptionally active virus. This is reinforced by the finding that p16 overexpression may be identified in OPSCC deemed negative for HPV by DNA in situ hybridization.[32] However, HPV can usually be confirmed by evaluation of E6 and E7 mRNA in a large proportion of these p16-overexpressing tumors.

It should be noted that there is substantial heterogeneity in HPV prevalence among studies, which is most likely due to different methods used for HPV detection (PCR, in-situ hybridization, Southern hybridization), the specific primers used for PCR, and sample source and collection methods (swabs, brushing, mouthwash, and biopsy).[14,22] The use of saliva-based assays has been proposed as a simple and rapid test for detecting HPV-HNSCC, but this remains to be validated.[17]

HUMAN PAPILLOMAVIRUS–ASSOCIATED OROPHARYNGEAL SQUAMOUS CELL CARCINOMA: DIAGNOSIS AND TREATMENT

For accurate diagnosis of HPV-OPSCC, the importance of thorough history-taking and physical examination, along with appropriate imaging, cannot be overemphasized.[12] An enlarged lateral neck mass may be noticed in asymptomatic patients, which often indicates metastasis to the lateral cervical lymph node. This occurs commonly in OPSCC because of its relatively late detection. As the tumor progresses, symptoms such as dysphasia or tonsillar pain may present. Precancerous lesions may not be easily visualized or palpable during routine dental examinations because of the preferred anatomic sites of HPV-OPSCC. Ultimately, only a tissue biopsy provides histopathologic confirmation of cancer. HPV status of the tumor can be revealed by PCR or immunohistochemical staining, as previously discussed.

There are now abundant data supporting the notion that HPV-OPSCC is a clinically distinct subset of HNSCC. HPV-OPSCC is associated with an overall better treatment outcome than non–HPV-OPSCC, with higher survival rate and lower adverse effects being reported.[2,35–38] In particular, HPV-OPSCC has shown a more favorable outcome when treated with radiation, either alone or with concomitant chemotherapy.[35,39] To this end, the 8th edition of the AJCC Staging Manual was published in the fall of 2016 with a major update to the clinical staging algorithm of high-risk HPV-OPSCC.[12] These changes are significantly different from staging criteria described in the 7th edition of the manual published in 2009.

In the current edition of the AJCC manual, HPV-OPSCCs are distinguished from non–HPV-OPSCCs. Clinical TNM (cTNM) and pathologic TNM (pTNM) are used to stage p16-positive, high-risk HPV-OPSCC. cTNM is applied to all patients with p16-positive, high-risk HPV-positive OPSCC, whereas pTNM is used only for patients who undergo surgery for their cancers.[12,40,41] An example of one of the striking changes is reflected in the reclassification of a p16-positive T1N2M0 cancer (2-cm tumor with 2 positive ipsilateral lymph nodes) from stage IV in the previous AJCC manual to stage I in the current iteration. Although some challenges exist, including potential difficulty of identifying the primary tumor site in advanced stage OPSCC and a lack of case-controlled studies, better prediction of HPV-OPSCC prognosis is expected using both the clinical and the pathologic data sets.[39]

The molecular mechanisms underlying the differences in treatment response between HPV-OPSCC and non–HPV-OPSCC remain unclear.[2,42] A recent study suggests that p16 sensitizes HPV-positive tumor cells to ionizing radiation by inhibiting homologous recombination-mediated DNA repair.[43] Although intriguing, the mechanisms enhancing survival of HPV-positive OPSCC remain to be more fully elucidated. With stratification of other risk factors such as tobacco use, further studies are necessary to achieve the optimal goal of personalizing therapeutics and providing more reliable prognostication for patients with HPV-OPSCC.[2,44] The interested reader is directed to Lydiatt and colleagues[12] for a full review of the changes in the 8th edition of the AJCC Cancer Staging Manual.

FUTURE STRATEGIES IN PREVENTION OF HUMAN PAPILLOMAVIRUS-ASSOCIATED HEAD AND NECK SQUAMOUS CELL CARCINOMA

The link between oral sex behavior and oropharyngeal HPV infection is evident. Strong association between orogenital contact and OPSCC was found in a hospital-based, case-control study of 100 newly diagnosed OPSCC patients and 200 controls.[45] A recent systematic review in 2014 found 50% to 80% of adolescents and young adults reported participation in oral sex.[46] Such widespread oral sexual practices among the young may be contributing to the rapid increase of OPSCC. To reduce HPV transmission, public health action has been taken with an emphasis on sexual behavior modification targeting the young, including recommending the use of condoms.[47] Although complete protection may not be possible, use of a condom has proven to be associated with reduced oral HPV transmission between sexual partners.

Currently, two Food and Drug Administration–approved HPV vaccines are available and recommended for girls and boys aged 9 through 14 years. Their effectiveness has been well established based on randomized trials.[48] The potential benefit of an HPV vaccine to reduce the increasing burden of HPV-OPSCC has been suggested.[22,47] Herrero and colleagues[49] published the results of the first randomized controlled trial demonstrating the benefit of HPV vaccination in preventing HPV-OPSCC in 2013. In their study, bivalent HPV vaccine showed a 93% vaccine efficacy in reducing oral HPV infection at 4-year follow-up. However, the efficacy of HPV vaccine for preventing head and neck cancer is still uncertain for several reasons including insufficient supporting data and low HPV vaccination coverage in men.[50] In addition, the association of OPSCC with other high-risk HPV types (other than 16 and 18), and synergism of HPV infection with environmental risk factors and chronic inflammation, also needs to be explored as a means of identifying potential therapeutic targets in patients who develop OPSCC, and as possible vaccine targets for prevention of HPV-OPSCC.[45]

SUMMARY

HPV-OPSCC is now recognized as a distinct subtype of HNSCC, and its recent increase in incidence is an emerging public health problem. This article reviewed the current understanding of HPV-OPSCC. Although the pathogenesis by which HPV infection in OPSCC remains incompletely understood, further investigations are necessary to reduce the global burden of OPSCC.

REFERENCES

1. Syrjanen K, Syrjanen S, Lamberg M, et al. Morphological and immunohistochemical evidence suggesting human papillomavirus (HPV) involvement in oral squamous cell carcinogenesis. Int J Oral Surg 1983;12(6):418–24.

2. Dayyani F, Etzel CJ, Liu M, et al. Meta-analysis of the impact of human papillomavirus (HPV) on cancer risk and overall survival in head and neck squamous cell carcinomas (HNSCC). Head Neck Oncol 2010;2:15.

3. Javadi P, Sharma A, Zahnd WE, et al. Evolving disparities in the epidemiology of oral cavity and oropharyngeal cancers. Cancer Causes Control 2017;28(6): 635–45.

4. Gillison ML, Chaturvedi AK, Anderson WF, et al. Epidemiology of human papillomavirus-positive head and neck squamous cell carcinoma. J Clin Oncol 2015;33(29):3235–42.

5. Patel MA, Blackford AL, Rettig EM, et al. Rising population of survivors of oral squamous cell cancer in the United States. Cancer 2016;122(9):1380–7.

6. Chaturvedi AK, Engels EA, Pfeiffer RM, et al. Human papillomavirus and rising oropharyngeal cancer incidence in the United States. J Clin Oncol 2011; 29(32):4294–301.

7. CDC Centers for Disease Control and Prevention: number of HPV-attributable cancer cases per year. Available at: https://www.cdc.gov/cancer/hpv/statistics/cases.htm. Accessed June 30, 2017.

8. Miller CS, Johnstone BM. Human papillomavirus as a risk factor for oral squamous cell carcinoma: a meta-analysis, 1982-1997. Oral Surg Oral Med Oral Pathol Oral Radiol Endod 2001;91(6):622–35.

9. Zafereo ME, Xu L, Dahlstrom KR, et al. Squamous cell carcinoma of the oral cavity often overexpresses p16 but is rarely driven by human papillomavirus. Oral Oncol 2016;56:47–53.

10. Huang CG, Lee LA, Liao CT, et al. Molecular and serologic markers of HPV 16 infection are associated with local recurrence in patients with oral cavity squamous cell carcinoma. Oncotarget 2017;8(21):34820–35.

11. El-Naggar AK, Chan JKC, Grandis JR, et al, editors. WHO classification of head and neck tumors. Lyon (France): IARC; 2017.

12. Lydiatt WM, Patel SG, O'Sullivan B, et al. Head and neck cancers-major changes in the American Joint Committee on Cancer Eighth Edition Cancer Staging Manual. CA Cancer J Clin 2017;67(2):122–37.

13. zur Hausen H. Papillomaviruses and cancer: from basic studies to clinical application. Nat Rev Cancer 2002;2(5):342–50.

14. Ragin CC, Modugno F, Gollin SM. The epidemiology and risk factors of head and neck cancer: a focus on human papillomavirus. J Dent Res 2007;86(2):104–14.

15. Saraiya M, Unger ER, Thompson TD, et al. US assessment of HPV types in cancers: implications for current and 9-valent HPV vaccines. J Natl Cancer Inst 2015; 107(6):djv086.

16. Doorbar J, Quint W, Banks L, et al. The biology and life-cycle of human papillomaviruses. Vaccine 2012;30(Suppl 5):F55–70.
17. Wasserman JK, Rourke R, Purgina B, et al. HPV DNA in saliva from patients with SCC of the head and neck is specific for p16-positive oropharyngeal tumours. J Otolaryngol Head Neck Surg 2017;46(1):3.
18. Ndiaye C, Mena M, Alemany L, et al. HPV DNA, E6/E7 mRNA, and p16INK4a detection in head and neck cancers: a systematic review and meta-analysis. Lancet Oncol 2014;15(12):1319–31.
19. International Agency for Research on Cancer: monographs on the evaluation of carcinogenic risks to humans. Updated 2009. Available at: http://monographs.iarc.fr/ENG/Monographs/vol100B/mono100B.pdf. Accessed June 30, 2017.
20. Viens LJ, Henley SJ, Watson M, et al. Human papillomavirus-associated cancers-United States, 2008-2012. MMWR Morb Mortal Wkly Rep 2016;65(26):661–6.
21. Mourad M, Jetmore T, Jategaonkar AA, et al. Epidemiological trends of head and neck cancer in the United States: a SEER population study. J Oral Maxillofac Surg 2017 [pii:S0278–2391(17)30537-2], [Epub ahead of print].
22. Chaturvedi AK, Anderson WF, Lortet-Tieulent J, et al. Worldwide trends in incidence rates for oral cavity and oropharyngeal cancers. J Clin Oncol 2013; 31(36):4550–9.
23. Hammarstedt L, Dahlstrand H, Lindquist D, et al. The incidence of tonsillar cancer in Sweden is increasing. Acta Otolaryngol 2007;127(9):988–92.
24. Chaturvedi AK, Engels EA, Anderson WF, et al. Incidence trends for human papillomavirus-related and -unrelated oral squamous cell carcinomas in the United States. J Clin Oncol 2008;26(4):612–9.
25. Heck JE, Berthiller J, Vaccarella S, et al. Sexual behaviours and the risk of head and neck cancers: a pooled analysis in the International Head and Neck Cancer Epidemiology (INHANCE) consortium. Int J Epidemiol 2010;39(1):166–81.
26. Zumsteg ZS, Cook-Wiens G, Yoshida E, et al. Incidence of oropharyngeal cancer among elderly patients in the United States. JAMA Oncol 2016;2(12):1617–23.
27. Lyford-Pike S, Peng S, Young GD, et al. Evidence for a role of the PD-1: PD-L1 pathway in immune resistance of HPV-associated head and neck squamous cell carcinoma. Cancer Res 2013;73(6):1733–41.
28. Chung CH, Zhang Q, Kong CS, et al. P16 protein expression and human papillomavirus status as prognostic biomarkers of nonoropharyngeal head and neck squamous cell carcinoma. J Clin Oncol 2014;32(35):3930–8.
29. Jordan RC, Lingen MW, Perez-Ordonez B, et al. Validation of methods for oropharyngeal cancer HPV status determination in US cooperative group trials. Am J Surg Pathol 2012;36(7):945–54.
30. Sedghizadeh PP, Billington WD, Paxton D, et al. Is p16-positive oropharyngeal squamous cell carcinoma associated with favorable prognosis? A systematic review and meta-analysis. Oral Oncol 2016;54:15–27.
31. Kouketsu A, Sato I, Abe S, et al. Detection of human papillomavirus infection in oral squamous cell carcinoma: a cohort study of Japanese patients. J Oral Pathol Med 2016;45(8):565–72.
32. Bishop JA, Ma XJ, Wang H, et al. Detection of transcriptionally active high-risk HPV in patients with head and neck squamous cell carcinoma as visualized by a novel E6/E7 mRNA in situ hybridization method. Am J Surg Pathol 2012; 36(12):1874–82.
33. Persson M, Brismar Wendel S, Ljungblad L, et al. High-risk human papillomavirus E6/E7 mRNA and L1 DNA as markers of residual/recurrent cervical intraepithelial neoplasia. Oncol Rep 2012;28(1):346–52.

34. Origoni M, Cristoforoni P, Carminati G, et al. E6/E7 mRNA testing for human papilloma virus-induced high-grade cervical intraepithelial disease (CIN2/CIN3): a promising perspective. Ecancermedicalscience 2015;9:533.

35. Ang KK, Harris J, Wheeler R, et al. Human papillomavirus and survival of patients with oropharyngeal cancer. N Engl J Med 2010;363(1):24–35.

36. Ang KK, Sturgis EM. Human papillomavirus as a marker of the natural history and response to therapy of head and neck squamous cell carcinoma. Semin Radiat Oncol 2012;22(2):128–42.

37. O'Rorke MA, Ellison MV, Murray LJ, et al. Human papillomavirus related head and neck cancer survival: a systematic review and meta-analysis. Oral Oncol 2012; 48(12):1191–201.

38. Udager AM, McHugh JB. Human papillomavirus-associated neoplasms of the head and neck. Surg Pathol Clin 2017;10(1):35–55.

39. Wang MB, Liu IY, Gornbein JA, et al. HPV-positive oropharyngeal carcinoma: a systematic review of treatment and prognosis. Otolaryngol Head Neck Surg 2015;153(5):758–69.

40. Amin MB, Greene FL, Edge SB, et al. The eighth edition AJCC Cancer Staging Manual: continuing to build a bridge from a population-based to a more "personalized" approach to cancer staging. CA Cancer J Clin 2017;67(2):93–9.

41. Pfister DG, Spencer S, Brizel DM, et al. Head and neck cancers, version 1.2015. J Natl Compr Canc Netw 2015;13(7):847–55 [quiz: 856].

42. Tribius S, Hoffmann M. Human papilloma virus infection in head and neck cancer. Dtsch Arztebl Int 2013;110(11):184–90, 190e1.

43. Dok R, Kalev P, Van Limbergen EJ, et al. p16INK4a impairs homologous recombination-mediated DNA repair in human papillomavirus-positive head and neck tumors. Cancer Res 2014;74(6):1739–51.

44. Kruger M, Pabst AM, Walter C, et al. The prevalence of human papilloma virus (HPV) infections in oral squamous cell carcinomas: a retrospective analysis of 88 patients and literature overview. J Craniomaxillofac Surg 2014;42(7):1506–14.

45. D'Souza G, Kreimer AR, Viscidi R, et al. Case-control study of human papillomavirus and oropharyngeal cancer. N Engl J Med 2007;356(19):1944–56.

46. Nguyen NP, Nguyen LM, Thomas S, et al. Oral sex and oropharyngeal cancer: the role of the primary care physicians. Medicine (Baltimore) 2016;95(28):e4228.

47. Odone A, Visciarelli S, Lalic T, et al. Human papillomavirus-associated cancers: a survey on otorhinolaryngologists' knowledge and attitudes on prevention. Acta Otorhinolaryngol Ital 2015;35(6):379–85.

48. Munoz N, Kjaer SK, Sigurdsson K, et al. Impact of human papillomavirus (HPV)-6/11/16/18 vaccine on all HPV-associated genital diseases in young women. J Natl Cancer Inst 2010;102(5):325–39.

49. Herrero R, Quint W, Hildesheim A, et al. Reduced prevalence of oral human papillomavirus (HPV) 4 years after bivalent HPV vaccination in a randomized clinical trial in Costa Rica. PLoS One 2013;8(7):e68329.

50. Han JJ, Beltran TH, Song JW, et al. Prevalence of genital human papillomavirus infection and human papillomavirus vaccination rates among US adult men: National Health And Nutrition Examination Survey (NHANES) 2013-2014. JAMA Oncol 2017;3(6):810–6.

Dental Treatment Planning for the Patient with Oral Cancer

Lauren E. Levi, DMD[a], Rajesh V. Lalla, DDS, PhD, DABOM[b],*

KEYWORDS

- Dental oncology • Oral cancer • Dental care for oral cancer
- Head and neck radiation therapy • Chemotherapy

KEY POINTS

- Treatment planning for a patient undergoing oral cancer therapy is crucial because it may help minimize a patient's risk for developing associated head and neck sequelae, which may halt a patient's oncologic therapy.
- Clinicians should ideally prepare a treatment plan and treat patients recently diagnosed with cancer before they undergo oncologic treatment.
- Clinicians should emphasize that patients should maintain excellent oral hygiene while undergoing cancer therapy.
- Obtaining a thorough medical and dental history is crucial because treatment planning considerations may change depending on a patient's medical history.

INTRODUCTION

Oral cancer therapy is associated with a multitude of head and neck sequelae that includes, but is not limited to, hyposalivation, increased risk for dental decay, radiation fibrosis syndrome, mucositis, chemotherapy-induced neuropathy, dysgeusia, dysphagia, mucosal lesions, and infections.[1–12] Preparing a detailed and comprehensive treatment plan for patients undergoing cancer therapy is essential to help minimize a patient's risk for developing these head and neck manifestations.[1–4] In addition to a comprehensive treatment plan, a detailed discussion reviewing the sequelae, oral hygiene instruction, and methods to help reduce risk for developing these conditions is necessary. This article discusses dental

Disclosure Statement: All authors declare that there are no financial conflicts associated with this study and that the funding source has no role in conceiving and performing the study.
[a] Department of Dentistry, Icahn School of Medicine at Mount Sinai, One Gustave L. Levy Place, Box 1187, New York, NY 10029, USA; [b] Department of Oral Medicine, UConn Health, 263 Farmington Avenue, Farmington, CT 06030-1605, USA
* Corresponding author.
E-mail address: Lalla@uchc.edu

dental.theclinics.com

treatment planning for the patient with oral cancer, including treating patients before therapy, those undergoing therapy, and those who have a history of oral cancer therapy.

PRETREATMENT INITIAL EXAMINATION

The ideal time to prepare a treatment plan for patients with oral cancer is before they have undergone therapy.[2,3] Oral cancer is often treated initially with surgery and subsequently with radiation therapy with or without concurrent chemotherapy, depending on the tumor location, stage, and grade.[1–4,13–15] Frequently, before undergoing head and neck radiation therapy with or without concurrent chemotherapy, patients are referred to a dental provider for a pretreatment dental evaluation.[1]

MEDICAL HISTORY

Obtaining a thorough medical history is crucial to the treatment planning process. Clinicians should not only review the patient's past medical history, past surgical history, medications, allergies, family history, and social history, but also record a detailed oncologic history. This oncologic history should include a history of any previous cancer and the associated treatment. This information is important because patients with a history of cancer therapy are at an increased risk for developing secondary cancers due to former cancer therapy, and thus they must be monitored closely for any recurrent or new lesions that may arise in their mouth.[4,16] In addition, certain dental procedures may be contraindicated in patients with a history of radiation therapy to the head and neck.[1–4] Furthermore, clinicians should discuss a patient's history of anti-resorptive and anti-angiogenic medications that may place the patient at risk for developing medication-related osteonecrosis of the jaw.[1–3,17] These medications include bisphosphonates, denosumab, bevacizumab, sunitinib, and potentially sorafenib.[2,3,17]

Previous History of Head and Neck Radiation Therapy

In addition to patients with head and neck cancer, patients with a history of lymphoma are often treated with head and neck radiation therapy.[3] Nonetheless, the cumulative dosage of patients with a history of lymphoma varies, and thus the dentist should discuss the patient's past radiation therapy with the patient's radiation oncologist.[18] Patients with a history of head and neck cancer often receive a cumulative dose of 50 to 70 Gy.[18] In addition, certain dental procedures may be contraindicated in patients with a history of radiation therapy to the head and neck.[1–3] For example, invasive dental procedures, especially procedures involving manipulation of the bone, are not recommended in areas of the mouth that have received high-dose radiation therapy.[1–4] High-dose radiation therapy is defined as a cumulative dose of greater than 50 Gy. Thus, in patients with a history of head and neck radiation therapy, clinicians should inquire about the cumulative radiation dosage and fractionation, the location of the radiation therapy, and the type of radiation therapy delivered. In addition, it is important to note that although patients may have received high-dose radiation therapy unilaterally, the contralateral anatomy may have received high-dose radiation as well. In other words, in a patient with a history of left base-of-tongue cancer who received unilateral left radiation, the right posterior mandibular teeth may have also received high-dose radiation therapy. Thus, the dental clinician must have a detailed discussion about the patient's head and neck radiotherapy not only with the patient but also with the patient's radiation oncologist.[1–3]

Oncologic History: Patient's Recent Diagnosis

Dental clinicians should have a detailed discussion with the patient and the patient's oncology team about the patient's recent oral cancer diagnosis, including the location of the tumor, the stage and grade, and proposed treatment.[1-3] For those patients undergoing head and neck radiation therapy, the dentist should inquire about the radiation commencement date as well as the date of the simulation. Ideally, all dental treatment should be completed before the simulation appointment.

Dental History

The clinician should review the patient's dental history and oral hygiene habits, including the date of the patient's last dental examination, prophylaxis, if indicated, and radiographs.[1] Radiographs taken within the last year should be reviewed.

ORAL EVALUATION
Extraoral Evaluation

Extraoral assessment should involve a cranial nerve examination, palpation of all muscles and soft tissues of the head and neck for lymphadenopathy, muscle tenderness, and any masses or abnormalities. In addition, clinicians should examine the skin of the head, neck, face, and scalp, document facial asymmetry, as well as take note of the patient's orientation to time, place, and level of alertness. In addition, clinicians should palpate the thyroid as well as the temporomandibular joint upon opening and closing. Maximum incisal opening, protrusion, and lateral excursions should be measured and recorded. Clinicians should also document trismus, the range of motion of the neck, and any TMJ abnormalities, including crepitus or evidence of disc displacement.[2]

Intraoral Evaluation

Intraoral examination should include not only a thorough evaluation of the dentition but also an assessment of the soft tissues of the oral cavity and oropharynx, including the mucosa, palatine tonsils, lingual tonsils, soft palate, uvula, hard palate, gingiva, lips, tongue, and floor of mouth.[1,2] In addition, health care professionals should palpate the submandibular, sublingual, and parotid glands and note salivary flow. Evaluation of the dentition should include a comprehensive hard tissue and periodontal evaluation, recording caries, missing teeth, signs of odontogenic or periodontal infection, and previous restorations. Percussion and palpation sensitivity along with tooth mobility should also be noted.[2,3]

Microbial Assessment

Active infections should be treated before the commencement of oncologic therapy and may require testing in order to determine the ideal course of treatment. Herpetic lesions such as herpes simplex are often diagnosed based on clinical presentation and treated with antiviral medications; however, certain presentations may require cytology smears for definitive diagnosis.[2-4,11,12] Intraoral draining fistulas or swelling may suggest a bacterial infection, and culturing of the lesions may aid in determining the ideal antibiotic. In addition, lesions that are suspicious for candida are often first treated upon clinical diagnosis with antifungal therapy; however, resistant lesions may be assessed with cytology smears, biopsy, or culture. Candidal infections may present as ulcerations at the corners of the mouth, the presence of a white plaque that can be removed with gauze (**Fig. 1**), a white lesion that cannot be removed, or an erythematous lesion most commonly on the tongue.[2,3,9,10]

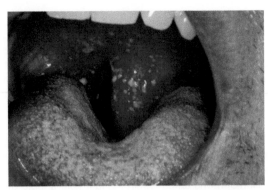

Fig. 1. Pseudomembranous candidiasis in a patient receiving radiation therapy for head and neck cancer. Note the white pseudomembranous lesions on the dorsal tongue, soft palate, uvula, and tonsillar pillar.

Imaging

Radiographic imaging is necessary to adequately diagnose caries, and thus clinicians should ideally take a full-mouth series of radiographs. Often, a panoramic radiograph or cone-beam computed tomography may be necessary if the treatment plan includes extractions and to provide a general assessment of the face.[2] Nonetheless, periapical and bitewing radiographs are often indicated for more detailed views of individual teeth for carious lesions. Images of the tumor volume and proposed treatment may be helpful in planning which teeth will be in the field of high-dose radiation.[2] Dentists should have a detailed discussion with the radiation oncologist about the proposed oncologic treatment plan and anatomy that will be affected by the radiation therapy.[1]

Additional Considerations for Head and Neck Radiation Patients

Clinicians might consider sialometry and sialochemistry in patients whose treatment plan includes head and neck radiation therapy. Establishing a baseline of salivary flow will allow for an objective measurement before the commencement of therapy. This measurement can then be compared with the salivary flow during and after therapy. Some clinicians may also consider measuring the pH of the saliva. An unstimulated whole salivary flow rate of less than 0.12 to 0.16 mL/min is considered low.[2]

PRETREATMENT OBJECTIVES

Although a thorough and comprehensive evaluation should be performed, dentists must be aware of the pretherapy dental objectives.[1–3] Patients recently diagnosed with oral cancer are often in need of emergent oncologic care, and thus the patient's treatment needs must be prioritized and triaged. Dental treatment objectives before oncologic therapy should be focused on eliminating oral conditions that may halt or interfere with a patient's oncologic therapy. Thus, clinicians should focus on eliminating sources of odontogenic or periodontal infection through extractions, scaling, and root planing or endodontic treatment. Nonrestorable carious teeth, teeth with hopeless periodontal involvement, or teeth with pulpal involvement with questionable prognosis that may require extensive treatment before commencement of chemotherapy or radiation should be extracted.[1,2] Extractions performed on patients who are undergoing head and neck radiation therapy should ideally be performed at least 2 weeks before commencement of radiation therapy to allow for epithelialization and wound healing.[2] Extractions should be performed as atraumatically as possible with primary closure without tissue tension.[2] Priority should be placed on teeth that are in the field of high-dose radiation therapy (>50 Gy). Odontogenic infections involving pulpal involvement in teeth that are restorable may be endodontically treated and sealed with a definitive restorative material, such as a resin or amalgam core. In addition to eliminating sources of infection, removing sources of trauma is an important treatment objective.[1–4] Restorations, fixed orthodontic appliances, or removable prostheses with jagged or rough edges that may elicit trauma should be adjusted because traumatic ulcerations may serve as a nidus for infections. In addition, pretreatment dental cleaning is recommended to help reduce the risk of oral mucositis.[2]

Radiation Mouth Guard Considerations

Patients undergoing head and neck radiation therapy who present with metal restorations are at risk of backscatter and forward scatter of radiation therapy.[2,19–23] Backscatter describes the phenomenon whereby the electrons in the metal restorations are liberated and move in a direction opposing the radiation beam. By contrast, forward scatter describes a similar phenomenon; however, the radioactive particles move in the same direction as the beam.[23] The intensity of scattering is proportional to the atomic number of the metal. Backscatter and forward scatter present a concern because dose enhancement and increased intensity of the beam are delivered to tissues adjacent to the metal restorations leading to an increased risk for developing oral mucositis.[2,19–23] As radiation therapy becomes more sophisticated, the dose distribution may be able to account for scatter; however, clinicians can fabricate radiation mouth guards to help combat the effects of backscatter and forward scatter.[2,19–23] A flexible mouth guard with a thickness in excess of 6 mm is recommended to create sufficient distance between the metal restorative material and the oral tissue.[2]

Patient Education

A detailed discussion reviewing the oral and dental sequelae associated with the patient's proposed treatment plan should occur between the dental clinician and the patient.[1–5]

Xerostomia/Hyposalivation

The dentist should review the risk for developing hyposalivation and xerostomia and explain that for patients undergoing high-dose radiation therapy involving the oral cavity, salivary composition and production will be irreversibly altered.[1–4] Salivary flow and composition may be temporarily altered by radiation doses as low as 10 Gy, whereas doses as low as 30 Gy may result in irreversible salivary gland changes.[3,4] Patients undergoing high-dose radiation therapy should be informed of the loss of the protective mechanisms of saliva to include saliva's role in deglutition, antimicrobial defense, speech, and preventing dental caries, thus leaving patients at an increased risk for developing dental decay.[1–4] In addition, dentists should inform patients that the salivary composition may change to become more viscous because serous acini are more radiosensitive.[4] A detailed discussion of oral hygiene instruction along with advocating that patients use a fluoridated toothpaste to brush their teeth at least twice daily is essential in addition to prescribing a high-strength fluoride dentifrice to be used nightly.[2–4] Furthermore, dental clinicians should educate patients about limiting sugar intake in between meals unless patients brush their teeth after consuming the sugar-laden snack or beverage.[4] Patients should also be discouraged from using alcoholic mouthwash given its desiccating effects.[2]

Radiation Fibrosis Syndrome and Trismus

Patients undergoing head and neck radiation therapy should be educated about the potential development of radiation fibrosis syndrome in the form of muscle tenderness, pain, and trismus.[2] The prevalence of trismus in patients with oral cancer has been reported to vary from 0% to 69%, and the wide range is thought to be due to method of trismus assessment, location of the tumor, tumor size, and the cancer treatment.[2–4,8,14,15,24] Symptoms of radiation fibrosis syndrome in patients with head and neck cancer include muscle tenderness, trismus, cervical dystonia, radiation-induced trigeminal neuralgia, lymphedema, dysarthria, and dysphagia.[24] Patients should be informed that radiation fibrosis syndrome is a late side effect of radiotherapy, and thus they should be encouraged to perform at-home exercises during and after the completion of radiation therapy.[24] These prophylactic exercises should be reviewed with patients before commencement of radiation therapy, and clinicians should encourage patients to complete these exercises daily throughout their lives.[4,24] In addition, clinicians should encourage patients to visit speech pathologists for swallowing therapy and physical therapists for prophylactic physical therapy.[1,2,4,24]

Osteoradionecrosis of the Jaw

A rare but serious manifestation of head and neck radiotherapy, osteoradionecrosis of the jaw (ORN), presents as an area of exposed bone in a previously irradiated area (**Fig. 2**).[2–4] The dentist should have a detailed discussion about a patient's risk for developing ORN and methods to help minimize the risk by advising patients against receiving invasive dental procedures in the field of high-dose therapy.[1–4]

Oral Mucositis

Oral mucositis refers to inflammation and ulceration of the oral mucosa as a side effect of chemotherapy or head and neck radiation therapy (**Fig. 3**). Clinicians should review the risks for developing oral mucositis in the setting of head and neck radiation therapy and chemotherapy.[1–7] Patients should be advised to rinse prophylactically with bland neutral rinses, such as solutions consisting of baking soda and salt water, and health care professionals should emphasize the importance of maintaining oral hygiene throughout their cancer treatment.[1–5] Furthermore, patients must be educated that maintaining oral hygiene is essential not only in aiding to reduce the severity of oral mucositis but also in preventing superinfection of mucositis by fungi or bacteria.[1–5]

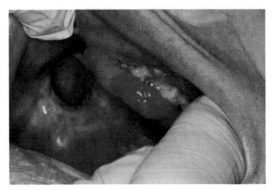

Fig. 2. ORN in a patient receiving radiation therapy for head and neck cancer. Note the exposed bone in the left maxilla and the surgical defect in the palate.

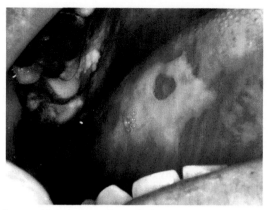

Fig. 3. A large oral mucositis lesion on the right lateral tongue of a patient receiving radiation therapy for head and neck cancer. Note the yellowish pseudomembrane covering much of the ulceration and the surrounding erythema.

Clinicians should educate patients about avoiding mouth rinses containing alcohol and hot or spicy foods.[1,3,4] Evidence-based clinical practice guidelines for the prevention and management of oral mucositis have been published.[6]

Oral Infections

Patients may develop oral infections during head and neck radiation therapy with or without concurrent chemotherapy.[1–4,9–12] Candidiasis is commonly seen in patients undergoing therapy and can result in dysphagia, dysgeusia, and in some cases, a burning sensation.[1–4,10,11] Patients should be informed of the risk of developing a fungal infection and be encouraged to visit a health care professional if they develop symptoms. In addition, patients should be informed of their increased risk for developing viral infections most commonly in the form of herpes viruses. Herpes viruses are frequently seen in immunocompromised patients.[1–4,11,12]

DENTAL TREATMENT PLANNING WHILE PATIENT IS UNDERGOING THERAPY

Special considerations should be taken for patients who present to the dentist while undergoing active oncologic therapy.

Patients Undergoing Head and Neck Radiation

Elective dental procedures should be avoided until after head and neck radiation therapy is complete. Nonetheless, in the event of an active infection, a discussion of the findings should be reviewed with the patient's oncologist to determine whether dental treatment can be performed during therapy. A detailed review of the risks and benefits of dental care along with risks for infection and other oral sequelae should be reviewed with the patient and the patient's oncology team.[1–4]

Patients Undergoing Chemotherapy

Elective dental procedures should be avoided in patients undergoing concurrent chemotherapy and radiation therapy ideally until patients have completed treatment.[1–4] Patients receiving active chemotherapy without radiation treatment may receive routine or necessary dental care when their counts are stable (absolute neutrophil count [ANC] at least 1000 cells/mm^3 and platelet count of at least 50,000 cells/mm^3).[1,3] Dentists should review the patient's chemotherapy schedule with the medical oncologist to coordinate dental care when the patient's counts will be stable. In addition, a complete blood count with differential should be ordered for patients the day of the proposed dental treatment to confirm that patient's ANC and platelet counts are stable.[2,3]

Chemotherapy-Induced Neurotoxicity/Neuropathy

Patients undergoing chemotherapy may complain of a throbbing pain in the absence of an odontogenic or periodontal cause. Certain chemotherapies associated with peripheral neuropathy may manifest in the jaw, whereas other chemotherapeutic agents, including plant-based vinca alkaloids, may cause neurotoxicity and present as throbbing jaw pain. Reviewing a patient's thorough medical history and a comprehensive evaluation with imaging are necessary for adequate diagnosis. Endodontic evaluation and pulp testing are important to help clinicians distinguish acute mandibular pain from neurotoxic or neuropathic-related pain, yet it is important to recognize that pulp testing may be altered in patients with neuropathic-related pain.[3,4]

DENTAL TREATMENT PLANNING AND MANAGEMENT AFTER PATIENT HAS COMPLETED THERAPY

Given the varied oral sequelae associated with head or neck radiation therapy and chemotherapy, patients should be encouraged to visit the dentist for frequent recall visits, which should include preventative care with topical fluoride applications.[1,2] These visits may help in reducing a patient's risk for developing the late side effects associated with head and neck radiation therapy as well as the severity of these conditions. A thorough and detailed discussion of oral hygiene is essential, including reviewing cariogenic dietary modifications and emphasizing the importance of using a fluoridated toothpaste. Patients who have undergone radiation therapy to the head and neck should be prescribed a fluoridated dentifrice with 1.1% neutral sodium fluoride to be used daily.[1,3,4]

Treatment of Nonrestorable Teeth

A patient with a history of radiation to the head and neck who presents with nonrestorable teeth should be treated with special attention to minimize his or her risk for developing ORN of the jaw. A detailed discussion with the patient's oncology team is essential to determine location of radiation delivered, type of radiation delivered, and dosing.[1] Teeth that are in the field of high-dose radiation therapy should be treated conservatively to minimize the patient's risk for developing ORN. Thus, if possible, endodontic therapy and a coronectomy or definitive restoration may be indicated.

If extractions are necessary, the specific doses to the areas of extraction should be determined because most cases of ORN occur at doses greater than 60 Gy. The site should also be considered because the posterior mandible is at greater risk for ORN. Surgical trauma and bone manipulation should be minimized, and primary closure is preferable. Other measures that have been studied to reduce the risk of ORN in irradiated bone include the use of prophylactic antibiotics, the use of hyperbaric oxygen before and after the extractions, and more recently, the use of pentoxifylline and tocopherol.[25]

MAXILLOFACIAL PROSTHETIC CONSIDERATIONS

Head, neck, and oral cancers often require surgical treatment, which is dictated by the tumor volume, location, size, and depth of infiltration.[18] Surgical resections of head and neck tumors, including maxillectomies, may necessitate fabrication of maxillofacial prosthetics, including palatal obturators, nasal prostheses, orbitals, or oculars. Maxillectomies may result in oro-antral communications; palatal obturators restore the floor of the nasal cavity as well as the roof of the oral cavity, aiding in deglutition and speech.[1] Ideally, resections that may require maxillofacial prosthetic appliances, such as palatal obturators, should be planned with that patient's oncology team before the patient undergoes surgery.[1] This not only allows the dentist to create diagnostic models on which the surgical plan can be delineated for fabrication of a surgical palatal obturator but also provides the dentist with treatment planning considerations for the interim obturator and for the patient's definitive restorative treatment plan. Similar considerations can be established for the fabrication of nasal, orbital, and ocular prostheses, and thus patients undergoing resections including the orbit or nose should visit the dentist before surgery.[1]

SUMMARY

Clinicians should be aware of the various treatment planning considerations in the management and evaluation of a patient undergoing oncologic therapy for oral cancer. By preparing a detailed and comprehensive treatment plan for patients undergoing cancer therapy, dentists can help minimize a patient's risk for developing these head and neck manifestations. In addition to a comprehensive treatment plan, a detailed discussion reviewing the sequelae, oral hygiene instruction, and methods to help reduce risk for developing these conditions is necessary.

REFERENCES

1. Harrison LB, et al. Head and neck cancer a multidisciplinary approach. Philadelphia: Wolters Kluwer/Lippincott-Raven; 2014.

2. Davies A, Epstein J. Oral complications of cancer and its management. Oxford (United Kingdom): Oxford University Press; 2010.

3. Oral Complications of Chemotherapy and Head/Neck Radiation. National Cancer Institute. 2016. Available at: https://www.cancer.gov/about-cancer/treatment/side-effects/mouth-throat/oral-complications-hp-pdq#section/_1. Accessed May 12, 2017.

4. Epstein JB, Thariat J, Bensadoun RJ, et al. Oral complications of cancer and cancer therapy. CA Cancer J Clin 2012;62(6):400–22.

5. Keefe DM, Schubert MM, Elting LS, et al. Updated clinical practice guidelines for the prevention and treatment of mucositis. Cancer 2007;109(5):820–31.

6. Lalla RV, Bowen J, Barasch A, et al. MASCC/ISOO clinical practice guidelines for the management of mucositis secondary to cancer therapy. Cancer 2014; 120(10):1453–61.

7. Trotti A, Bellm LA, Epstein JB, et al. Mucositis incidence, severity and associated outcomes in patients with head and neck cancer receiving radiotherapy with or without chemotherapy: a systematic literature review. Radiother Oncol 2003; 66(3):253–62.

8. Dijkstra PU, Kalk WW, Roodenburg JL. Trismus in head and neck oncology: a systematic review. Oral Oncol 2004;40(9):879–89.

9. Lalla RV, Latortue MC, Hong CH, et al. A systematic review of oral fungal infections in patients receiving cancer therapy. Support Care Cancer 2010;18(8): 985–92.

10. Bensadoun RJ, Patton LL, Lalla RV, et al. Oropharyngeal candidiasis in head and neck cancer patients treated with radiation: update 2011. Support Care Cancer 2011;19(6):737–44.
11. Epstein JB, Gorsky M, Hancock P, et al. The prevalence of herpes simplex virus shedding and infection in the oral cavity of seropositive patients undergoing head and neck radiation therapy. Oral Surg Oral Med Oral Pathol Oral Radiol Endod 2002;94(6):712–6.
12. Samonis G, Mantadakis E, Maraki S, et al. Orofacial viral infections in the immunocompromised host. Oncol Rep 2000;7(6):1389–94.
13. Shah JP, Gil Z. Current concepts in management of oral cancer-surgery. Oral Oncol 2009;45(4–5):394–401.
14. Bertrand J, Luc B, Philippe M, et al. Anterior mandibular osteotomy for tumor extirpation: a critical evaluation. Head Neck 2000;22(4):323–7.
15. Eisen MD, Weinstein GS, Chalian A, et al. Morbidity after midline mandibulotomy and radiation therapy. Am J Otolaryngol 2000;21(5):312–7.
16. Abeloff MD. Abeloff's clinical oncology. Philadelphia: Churchill Livingstone/Elsevier; 2014.
17. Ruggiero SL, Dodson TB, Fantasia J, et al. American Association of Oral and Maxillofacial Surgeons position paper on medication-related osteonecrosis of the jaw–2014 update. J Oral Maxillofac Surg 2014;72(10):1938–56.
18. Lee NY, Lu JJ. Target volume delineation and field setup: a practical guide for conformal and intensity-modulated radiation therapy. Heidelberg (Germany): Springer; 2013.
19. Wang R, Boyle A. A convenient method for guarding against localized mucositis during radiation therapy. J Prosthodont 1994;3:198–201.
20. Allan E, et al. Dosimetric verification of dental stent efficacy in head and neck radiation therapy using modern radiation therapy techniques: quality of life (QOL) and treatment compliance implications. Int J Radiat Oncol Biol Phys 2016; 94(4):875–6.
21. Katsura K, Utsunomiya S, Abe E, et al. A study on a dental device for the prevention of mucosal dose enhancement caused by backscatter radiation from dental alloy during external beam radiotherapy. J Radiat Res 2016;57(6):709–13. Available at: www.ncbi.nlm.nih.gov/pmc/articles/PMC5137298/. Accessed May 9, 2017.
22. Chin DWH, Treister N, Friedland B, et al. Effect of dental restorations and prostheses on radiotherapy dose distribution: a Monte Carlo Study. J Appl Clin Med Phys 2009;10(1):2853.
23. Karakoyun-Celik O, Norris CM Jr, Tishler R, et al. Definitive radiotherapy with interstitial implant boost for squamous cell carcinoma of the tongue base. Head Neck 2005;27(5):353–61.
24. Frontera WR, et al. Essentials of physical medicine and rehabilitation: musculoskeletal disorders, pain, and rehabilitation. Philadelphia: Saunders/Elsevier; 2015.
25. Nabil S, Samman N. Incidence and prevention of osteoradionecrosis after dental extraction in irradiated patients: a systematic review. Int J Oral Maxillofac Surg 2011;40(3):229–43.

Dental Management of Patients Who Have Undergone Oral Cancer Therapy

Alessandro Villa, DDS, PhD, MPH[a,b],
Sunday O. Akintoye, BDS, DDS, MS[c,*]

KEYWORDS

- Oral mucositis • Xerostomia • Infections • Tissue fibrosis • Trismus
- Osteoradionecrosis

KEY POINTS

- Patients undergoing treatment of oral cancer may experience short-term and long-term oral cavity complications.
- The most common side effects from oral cancer therapy include mucositis, infections, and osteoradionecrosis of the jaws.
- Effective dental management of patients with oral cancer involves the coordination of care among several health care professionals.

INTRODUCTION

Oral cancers remain a major health concern worldwide. The tumor-related and patient-related factors, as well as treatment complications, negatively affect the 5-year survival rate and quality of life of survivors.[1] The common treatment modalities for oral cancer include surgery, radiotherapy, chemotherapy, or a combination of these depending on the tumor type, anatomic site, and stage of the cancer. Chemotherapeutic drugs are associated with a wide spectrum of hematologic toxicities that include anemia, leukopenia, neutropenia, and thrombocytopenia.[2] Although immunosuppression in patients with oral cancer is usually transient, these patients are still susceptible to a high risk of bacterial, viral, and fungal infections. The major objectives of oral cancer therapies are complete tumor control, with minimal treatment complications and improved

Disclosures: None.
[a] Department of Oral Medicine, Infection, and Immunity, Harvard School of Dental Medicine, 188 Longwood Avenue, Boston, MA 02115, USA; [b] Division of Oral Medicine and Dentistry, Brigham and Women's Hospital, 1620 Tremont Street, Suite BC3-028, Boston, MA 02118, USA; [c] Department of Oral Medicine, University of Pennsylvania School of Dental Medicine, Robert Schattner Room 211, 240 South 40th Street, Philadelphia, PA 19104, USA
* Corresponding author.
E-mail address: akintoye@upenn.edu

Dent Clin N Am 62 (2018) 131–142
http://dx.doi.org/10.1016/j.cden.2017.08.010
0011-8532/18/© 2017 Elsevier Inc. All rights reserved.

quality of life. However, acute and long-term toxicities associated with treatment may decrease patients' tolerance to therapy, leading to a change in treatment schedules. Ultimately, suboptimal treatment schedules translate into poor patient outcomes, increased days of hospitalization, and increased health care costs.[3–5] Early complications of oral cancer therapies can result from acute toxic effects of radiotherapy and chemotherapy affecting several orofacial structures. These complications may present as oropharyngeal and gastrointestinal mucositis, salivary gland hypofunction, odontogenic infections, pain, and neurotoxicity. Late complications often take months or years to develop, and include orofacial soft tissue fibrosis, trismus, osteoradionecrosis (ORN), and cancer recurrence.[6] These complications are also associated with significant loss of function and facial disfigurement that lead to diminished quality of life and unwanted psychosocial outcomes.[7] Considering the dose-limiting effects and patient outcomes that result from treatment toxicities, it is essential that management of patients with oral cancer involves a multidisciplinary team of health care professionals that includes medical and dental health care providers as well as social workers and nutrition specialists.[5] Prompt diagnosis, treatment planning, and judicious provision of dental care before, during, and after oral cancer therapy are essential aspects of management that may enhance oral cancer survivorship and lead to improved quality of life.[8]

DENTAL MANAGEMENT CONSIDERATIONS IN ORAL CANCER MANAGEMENT

Although oral complications of chemotherapy are limited to a few weeks, the effects of radiotherapy tend to persist for months to years. The combination of surgery with chemoradiotherapy can further exacerbate these complications. It is prudent to consider the impact of treatment complications on all orofacial structures so that dental treatment can be provided effectively (**Table 1**).

Skin

The incidence of acute dermatitis in patients with oral cancer receiving radiotherapy can be as high as 95% because of high radiation doses to the skin and the combined effects of chemoradiotherapy.[9] Oral cancer therapies promote an imbalance in the activities of proinflammatory and profibrotic cytokines in the skin causing vascular damage and decreased blood perfusion. These effects may result in orofacial skin ulceration and necrosis.[10] The patient's medical history combined with clinical appearance make the diagnosis of radiation dermatitis straightforward. It is vital to prevent and control acute dermatitis as much as possible so that the radiochemotherapeutic regimen is uninterrupted. Avoiding unnecessary skin irradiation is the best preventive approach to minimizing the occurrence of radiation dermatitis. Chronic skin ulceration and infected wounds require special dressings that promote healing. Surgical care combined with skin grafting may be necessary when extensive necrosis has already set in. The use of low-intensity laser therapy may be beneficial to improve vascularization and promote healing in the damaged skin.[11] More recently, the administration of glutamine to promote protein synthesis and cell proliferation has been found to be an effective therapy for radiation dermatitis.[12]

Oral Mucosa

Oral cancer therapies can cause oral mucositis, an acute reaction characterized by erythema, mucosal ulceration, oropharyngeal pain, and speech difficulties (**Fig. 1**). Radiation-induced oral mucositis develops when radiation doses exceed 30 Gy. The frequency of oral mucositis secondary to chemotherapy ranges from 20% to 40%, and the incidence is 50% for those patients who receive induction

Table 1
Complications associated with oral cancer therapies

Affected Structures	Potential Outcomes of Chemotherapy, Radiotherapy, and Surgery
Skin	Radiation dermatitis
Oral mucosa	Mucositis Infections: fungal, viral, bacterial
Teeth	Caries caused by hyposalivation
Jaws/bone	Chemotoxicity Osteoradionecrosis Secondary infections Mastication difficulties
Salivary glands	Hyposalivation/xerostomia
Muscles and soft tissues	Fibrosis Mastication Dysphagia Speech difficulties
Temporomandibular joint	Fibrosis and trismus
Tongue and taste buds	Taste dysfunction
Others	Pain Dentofacial abnormalities Altered quality of life

Modified from Turner L, Mupparapu M, Akintoye SO. Review of the complications associated with treatment of oropharyngeal cancer: a guide for the dental practitioner. Quintessence Int 2013;44(3):267–79.

chemotherapy.[13,14] Methotrexate, cyclophosphamide, cisplatin, and 5-fluorouracil are associated with the highest risk for mucositis. The first signs of mucositis typically begin 3 to 4 days following the administration of the chemotherapeutic drug and last for about 15 days. Patients complain of oral sensitivity and burning, which are followed by the formation of painful ulcers.[8,15] The risks of developing mucositis depend on the chemotherapy cycle, whereas the severity of mucositis increases with the intensity of therapy.[8,15]

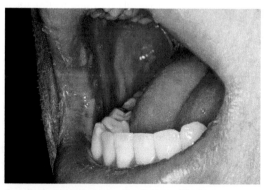

Fig. 1. Mucositis after radiation therapy. Oral mucositis in a young male patient with nasopharyngeal rhabdomyosarcoma after radiotherapy.

Preventive strategies used to attenuate the severity of oral mucositis secondary to oral cancer therapy include maintenance of optimal oral hygiene and the implementation of oral care protocols. Rinsing the mouth frequently with 0.9% saline or sodium bicarbonate and meticulous daily tooth brushing and flossing decrease bacterial colonization of the oral ulcers and therefore shorten the ulcer healing time.[5,16,17] Ill-fitting dentures and orthodontic appliances that have the potential to cause local trauma to the mouth should be adjusted or removed.[5]

Oral cryotherapy for 30 minutes is a recommended preventive measure in patients receiving boluses of 5-fluorouracil chemotherapy.[16] Also, benzydamine hydrochloride oral rinse effectively reduces the severity of oral mucositis based on its antiinflammatory properties in patients with oral cancer treated with less than 50-Gy doses of radiotherapy.[16] More recent evidence indicates that patients treated with doses greater than 50 Gy still benefit from the antiinflammatory properties of benzydamine hydrochloride.[18] The only medication approved for mucositis by the US Food and Drug Administration (FDA) is palifermin (keratinocyte growth factor). Palifermin is not used in oral cancer settings. It is used more appropriately to treat mucositis secondary to conditioning regimens in bone marrow transplant patients.[19] Similarly, low-level laser therapy (LLLT) or photobiomodulation has been used with promising results in hematopoietic stem cell transplants patients receiving high-dose chemotherapy, but it is not recommended for the treatment of chemoradiation-induced mucositis.[20,21] Laser light promotes angiogenesis; stimulates the production of serotonin, collagen, and cortisol; and increases DNA and RNA synthesis and cellular metabolism.[22] As such, LLLT may negatively affect tumor behaviors or increase resistance to oral cancer therapy. Several agents are recommended for pain management in patients with mucositis, although their efficacy remains unclear. These agents include palliative rinses such as MuGard (AMAG Pharmaceuticals Inc, Waltham, MA), Episil (Camurus AB, Lund, Sweden), Caphosol (EUSA Pharma Ltd, Hemel Hempstead, United Kingdom), GelClair (Alliance Pharma plc, Wiltshire, United Kingdom), and Magic mouthwash (also called Miracle mouthwash).[23–28] Application of petroleum-based or lanolin-based lip care products may help to minimize tissue injury by reducing lip dryness.

Teeth

Any tooth in the irradiated field during oral cancer therapy is at risk of developing radiation caries, which can rapidly progress to periapical disease.[17] Also, chemotherapy can exacerbate any subclinical dental disorder. In addition to the direct effects of radiation on the teeth, a decrease in salivary flow and shift of the oral microbial flora to a more cariogenic type are additional factors that promote advanced dental caries.[5,17] A common recommendation is to conduct complete dental and radiographic evaluations and provide urgent dental treatments before oral cancer therapy commences.[29–31] However, timing of cancer therapy and patient conditions are often suboptimal to allow these to be completed. In addition to these management constraints, the clinical criteria for selecting restorable and nonrestorable teeth are not clear-cut but are based on sound clinical judgment and experience of the dental care provider.[29–32] When practicable, teeth with advanced carious lesions, periapical disorders, and periodontal infections may need to be extracted so that they do not precipitate dental complications and infections during oral cancer therapy. Patients who have neglected their dental care and who present with poor oral hygiene and multiple unrestorable dental lesions require a less conservative dental management approach, such as multiple tooth extractions, before cancer therapy. To prevent or slow down the rate/progression of dental caries, the use of 0.12% to 0.2%

chlorhexidine mouth rinse helps reduce the count of cariogenic bacteria, and application of topical fluoride such as 1.1% neutral sodium fluoride or a 0.4% stannous fluoride retards tooth demineralization.[5,17] Improving salivary flow with pharmacologic and nonpharmacologic agents reduces oral microbial counts and promotes tooth remineralization.

Jaws/Bone

The jaw bones are usually within the radiation field during oral cancer radiotherapy, resulting in the potential complication of ORN of the jaws (**Fig. 2**).[2] ORN presents clinically as a painful or painless nonhealing bone exposure within the irradiated field. On histopathology, ORN shows the classic features of a radiation-induced hypoxic-hypovascular-hypocellular tissue.[33,34] Several reports have placed the incidence of jaw ORN between 2.6% and 44%. A lower ORN incidence is attributed to the maxilla because it is more vascular and less corticated than the mandible. Patients who receive radiation doses greater than 50 Gy to the head and neck region are highly susceptible to ORN.[5,33] Although the early cellular events associated with radiation damage to bone begin with the first 2 weeks, ORN is considered a late complication of radiotherapy because it may not present clinically for several months.[5,34] Trauma from dental extractions or any other dental surgical procedure in the affected jaw bone provides a portal of entry for oral microbes, which can further advance the osteoradionecrotic process.

Diagnosis and management of ORN are based on patient's history and clinical presentation combined with radiological and histopathologic tests. Treatment is also guided by the extent of bone exposure and severity of symptoms.[5] Treatment can range from conservative therapy with antibiotics and saline irrigation to surgical debridement and flap surgery. Several protocols have incorporated the use of hyperbaric oxygen (HBO) therapy as adjunctive therapy before and after surgical treatment of ORN to promote healing.[35,36] Reports on the effectiveness of HBO therapy remain controversial and HBO therapy is not recommended in patients with metastatic cancers because of its angiogenic property.[37]

Salivary Glands

Any of the 3 major salivary glands (especially the parotid glands) and the numerous minor salivary glands may be within the radiation field during oral cancer radiotherapy. The salivary gland parenchyma is sensitive to radiation damage and toxic

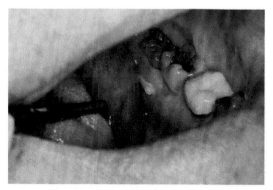

Fig. 2. Osteoradionecrosis. Mandibular osteoradionecrosis of the left mylohyoid ridge in a patient after radiation therapy for the head and neck.

effects of chemotherapy. This damage results in a significant reduction in the flow of saliva, so patients develop xerostomia and other signs and symptoms of oral dryness (**Fig. 3**). About 50% to 60% of patients undergoing oral cancer therapy present with salivary gland hypofunction.[38] The reduced salivary flow translates to a marked reduction in the physiologic, biochemical, and antimicrobial functions of saliva within the oral cavity, which has negative effects on mastication, deglutition, olfaction, and oral functions and diminish the patient's overall health status and quality of life.[36] Patients with oral cancer are also more susceptible to rapidly advancing dental caries caused by the loss of the remineralizing functions of saliva; a higher number of teeth develop dental caries and periodontal diseases because of loss of the antimicrobial functions of saliva.[36] The loss of salivary functions coupled with chemotherapy-induced immunosuppression in patients with oral cancer further exacerbate the severity of oral infections. The use of fractionated radiation, intensity-modulated radiation therapy that narrows the irradiated area and administration of the radioprotective drug, amifostine, are effective ways to minimize radiation-induced salivary gland damage.[39] Both pharmacologic and nonpharmacologic approaches have been used successfully to alleviate the effects of reduced salivary flow. Dissolving sugarless lozenges or chewing sugarless gums can stimulate residual salivary gland acini to secrete more saliva. Sucking on ice cubes or sugarless popsicles may help by keeping the mouth cool and moist. Systemic sialagogues, such as pilocarpine and cevimeline, are cholinergic agonists that are effective in improving salivary flow from residual salivary acini.[40] Saliva substitutes (such as Biotene products) used to lubricate the oral mucosa are well tolerated by most patients but they have limited effects because they do not restore the biochemical and antimicrobial properties of saliva.[41] As previously stated, the increased oral microbial load caused by hyposalivation drastically increases the patient's dental plaque and caries indices. Therefore, application of topical fluoride is an effective way to mitigate the high susceptibility to dental caries.[5,17] Alternative and newer therapies, such as acupuncture and stem cell therapy, are currently being explored to improve hyposalivation associated with oral cancer therapies.[42]

Muscles of Mastication and Temporomandibular Joint

Radiotherapy to the head and neck region can be complicated by fibrosis of the muscles of mastication and degenerative changes in the temporomandibular joints. These changes present as trismus characterized by reduced mouth opening caused by

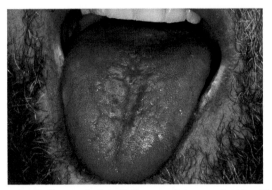

Fig. 3. Oral dryness. Radiotherapy-induced dry mouth is associated with depapillation of tongue dorsum and hairy tongue.

limited contraction of the muscles of mastication (**Fig. 4**). Trismus begins within the first 3 days of radiation therapy and the patient may not be aware of the gradual reduction in mouth opening until it becomes associated with pain or significant dysfunction. Surgical therapy for oral cancer with or without radiotherapy can cause scar tissue formation and nerve damage that further limit the full range of motion of the temporomandibular joint. Also, the severity of trismus often correlates with increased radiation doses; the cumulative effect of radiation is especially pronounced in patients who have previously received radiotherapy to the same orofacial region.[43] Trismus has significant impact on mastication, talking, ability to maintain optimum oral hygiene, as well as ability to receive dental care because of limited access to the oral cavity. Patients who develop trismus have compromised nutritional status that can hinder postoperative healing of orofacial structures and quality of life. The risks of trismus should always be considered during the preradiotherapy planning phase. The radiation dose to the masticatory apparatus should be minimized as much as possible without compromising locoregional tumor control. Radiotherapy-induced trismus is challenging to manage. Any limitation in temporomandibular joint mobility can trigger disuse atrophy of the muscles of mastication, which further exacerbates the trismus. Therefore, commencing jaw stretching exercises before trismus sets in is an effective preventive approach.[44] Continuous use of passive stretching exercises during the postradiotherapy period prevents tonic muscle contraction and improves mandibular opening.[45] Improving trismus with flap surgery and medications, such as botulinum toxin injections and pentoxifylline, are other treatment approaches that are being explored.[44,46]

Tongue and Taste Buds

Patients with oral cancer may report taste changes (dysgeusia) after chemotherapy as well as metallic or chemical taste during the administration of chemotherapy.[47] Similarly, radiation as low as 2 to 4 Gy to the oral mucosa can compromise taste perception.[4,48] Patients may complain of a lack of taste (ageusia), reduced taste sensitivity (hypogeusia), or heightened sensitivity (hypergeusia). Any of these taste changes can have profound effects on nutrition, leading to weight loss and overall poor quality of life.[38] Chemotherapeutic drugs target cells with a high mitotic activity and may damage taste receptors. In addition, several chemotherapeutic agents secreted in saliva cause a direct damage to taste receptors. Generalized oral dryness secondary to

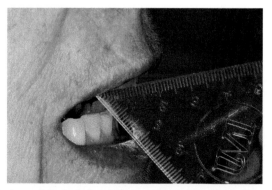

Fig. 4. Trismus. Maximum interincisal mouth opening was limited to 9 mm in this female patient who received radiotherapy to the head and neck.

radiation and chemotherapy may also lead to dysgeusia.[49,50] However, taste changes are often temporary, lasting only a few months.

Neurotoxicity and Pain

Neurotoxicity and neuropathic pain are self-limiting adverse effects secondary to oral cancer therapies.[51] Common symptoms of neurotoxicity include fatigue, neuropathy, and altered cognitive function.[52] Little is known about the mechanism of chemotherapy-induced neurotoxicity, although inflammation, oxidative stress, and DNA damage have been implicated.[53] Oral cancer surgery can also disturb adjacent nerves in the surgical field to cause oral neuropathic pain.[54] Extensive ORN can also cause paresthesia/anesthesia, making the patient uncomfortable. Treatment depends on the severity of the symptoms and centers on pain control with opioids as the first-line therapy. Other drugs used to treat chemotherapy-induced neurotoxicity include anticonvulsants, antidepressants, corticosteroids, and anesthetics, as well as nutritional supplementation with alpha-lipoic acid, vitamin E, erythropoietin, and acetyl-L-carnitine.[55–59]

Oral Infections

Chemotherapy-induced myelosuppression, development of oral mucositis, hyposalivation, and poor oral hygiene alter oral microbial flora and increase oral microbial load, making the patients susceptible to opportunistic bacterial, viral, and fungal infections.[48,60,61] The patients have a higher risk of developing odontogenic infections if they do not receive prompt care for any dental or periodontal disorder. However, candidal infection is the most common oral infection (**Fig. 5**). Patients can present with extensive pseudomembranous or erythematous coating on any of the mucosal surfaces. Although topical antifungal therapy may be effective in controlling oral candidiasis in some patients, systemic antifungal therapy is often necessary in cases of disseminated oral candidiasis and other fungal infections, like aspergillosis and mucormycosis.[5,30]

It is very likely that patients with oral cancer have been exposed to herpes simplex virus (HSV) at an earlier age. Therefore, HSV infections can be reactivated by chemotherapy-induced myelosuppression, making the patient develop vesicular eruptions and shallow ulcerations on both keratinized and nonkeratinized oral mucosa (**Fig. 6**). The use of prophylactic antiviral therapy with acyclovir is often advocated in patients who are seropositive for HSV.[5,30]

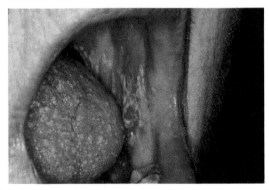

Fig. 5. Oral candidiasis. Pseudomembranous candidiasis in a patient with head and neck cancer after radiotherapy.

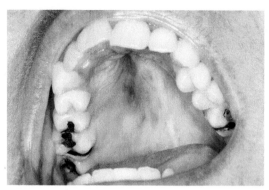

Fig. 6. Recrudescent HSV infection in a patient with chemotherapy-induced myelosuppression.

SUMMARY

Effective dental management of patients with oral cancer involves the coordination of care among several health care professionals. Oral health care assessment, including clinical and radiological evaluations of the orofacial complex, should be performed before oral cancer therapy. Prophylactic therapies and control dental conditions that can otherwise hinder the provision of optimal cancer therapies must be considered before initiation of cancer treatment. In addition, maintenance of good oral hygiene and provision of appropriate dental care during the therapy and after the therapy for oral cancer may alleviate oral pain and discomfort and help establish an enhanced quality of life for survivors.

REFERENCES

1. Edwards BK, Howe HL, Ries LA, et al. Annual report to the nation on the status of cancer, 1973-1999, featuring implications of age and aging on U.S. cancer burden. Cancer 2002;94(10):2766–92.

2. Buglione M, Cavagnini R, Di Rosario F, et al. Oral toxicity management in head and neck cancer patients treated with chemotherapy and radiation: dental pathologies and osteoradionecrosis (Part 1) literature review and consensus statement. Crit Rev Oncol Hematol 2016;97:131–42.

3. Schmitz S, Ang KK, Vermorken J, et al. Targeted therapies for squamous cell carcinoma of the head and neck: current knowledge and future directions. Cancer Treat Rev 2014;40(3):390–404.

4. Watters AL, Epstein JB, Agulnik M. Oral complications of targeted cancer therapies: a narrative literature review. Oral Oncol 2011;47(6):441–8.

5. Turner L, Mupparapu M, Akintoye SO. Review of the complications associated with treatment of oropharyngeal cancer: a guide for the dental practitioner. Quintessence Int 2013;44(3):267–79.

6. Villa A, Sonis S. Toxicities associated with head and neck cancer treatment and oncology-related clinical trials. Curr Probl Cancer 2016;40(5–6):244–57.

7. Rudat V, Wannenmacher M. Role of multimodal treatment in oropharynx, larynx, and hypopharynx cancer. Semin Surg Oncol 2001;20(1):66–74.

8. Sonis ST. Oral mucositis in head and neck cancer: risk, biology, and management. Am Soc Clin Oncol Educ Book 2013.

9. Singh M, Alavi A, Wong R, et al. Radiodermatitis: a review of our current understanding. Am J Clin Dermatol 2016;17(3):277–92.

10. Spalek M. Chronic radiation-induced dermatitis: challenges and solutions. Clin Cosmet Investig Dermatol 2016;9:473–82.

11. Schindl A, Schindl M, Pernerstorfer-Schon H, et al. Low intensity laser irradiation in the treatment of recalcitrant radiation ulcers in patients with breast cancer—long-term results of 3 cases. Photodermatol Photoimmunol Photomed 2000; 16(1):34–7.

12. Lopez-Vaquero D, Gutierrez-Bayard L, Rodriguez-Ruiz JA, et al. Double-blind randomized study of oral glutamine on the management of radio/chemotherapy-induced mucositis and dermatitis in head and neck cancer. Mol Clin Oncol 2017;6(6):931–6.

13. Sonis ST. The pathobiology of mucositis. Nat Rev Cancer 2004;4(4):277–84.

14. Blijlevens N, Schwenkglenks M, Bacon P, et al. Prospective oral mucositis audit: oral mucositis in patients receiving high-dose melphalan or BEAM conditioning chemotherapy—European blood and marrow transplantation mucositis advisory group. J Clin Oncol 2008;26(9):1519–25.

15. Villa A, Sonis ST. Pharmacotherapy for the management of cancer regimen-related oral mucositis. Expert Opin Pharmacother 2016;17(13):1801–7.

16. Lalla RV, Bowen J, Barasch A, et al. MASCC/ISOO clinical practice guidelines for the management of mucositis secondary to cancer therapy. Cancer 2014; 120(10):1453–61.

17. Hong CH, Napenas JJ, Hodgson BD, et al. A systematic review of dental disease in patients undergoing cancer therapy. Support Care Cancer 2010;18(8): 1007–21.

18. Rastogi M, Khurana R, Revannasiddaiah S, et al. Role of benzydamine hydrochloride in the prevention of oral mucositis in head and neck cancer patients treated with radiotherapy (>50 Gy) with or without chemotherapy. Support Care Cancer 2017;25(5):1439–43.

19. Spielberger R, Stiff P, Bensinger W, et al. Palifermin for oral mucositis after intensive therapy for hematologic cancers. N Engl J Med 2004;351(25):2590–8.

20. Oberoi S, Zamperlini-Netto G, Beyene J, et al. Effect of prophylactic low level laser therapy on oral mucositis: a systematic review and meta-analysis. PLoS One 2014;9(9):e107418.

21. Sonis ST, Hashemi S, Epstein JB, et al. Could the biological robustness of low level laser therapy (photobiomodulation) impact its use in the management of mucositis in head and neck cancer patients. Oral Oncol 2016;54:7–14.

22. Basso FG, Oliveira CF, Kurachi C, et al. Biostimulatory effect of low-level laser therapy on keratinocytes in vitro. Lasers Med Sci 2013;28(2):367–74.

23. Allison RR, Ambrad AA, Arshoun Y, et al. Multi-institutional, randomized, double-blind, placebo-controlled trial to assess the efficacy of a mucoadhesive hydrogel (MuGard) in mitigating oral mucositis symptoms in patients being treated with chemoradiation therapy for cancers of the head and neck. Cancer 2014; 120(9):1433–40.

24. Buchsel PC. Polyvinylpyrrolidone-sodium hyaluronate gel (Gelclair): a bioadherent oral gel for the treatment of oral mucositis and other painful oral lesions. Expert Opin Drug Metab Toxicol 2008;4(11):1449–54.

25. Quinn B. Efficacy of a supersaturated calcium phosphate oral rinse for the prevention and treatment of oral mucositis in patients receiving high-dose cancer therapy: a review of current data. Eur J Cancer Care 2013;22(5):564–79.

26. Raphael MF, den Boer AM, Kollen WJ, et al. Caphosol, a therapeutic option in case of cancer therapy-induced oral mucositis in children? Results from a prospective multicenter double blind randomized controlled trial. Support Care Cancer 2014;22(1):3–6.

27. Yuan A, Sonis S. Emerging therapies for the prevention and treatment of oral mucositis. Expert Opin Emerg Drugs 2014;19(3):343–51.

28. Dodd MJ, Dibble SL, Miaskowski C, et al. Randomized clinical trial of the effectiveness of 3 commonly used mouthwashes to treat chemotherapy-induced mucositis. Oral Surg Oral Med Oral Pathol Oral Radiol Endod 2000;90(1):39–47.

29. National Institutes of Health Consensus Development Panel. Consensus statement: oral complications of cancer therapies. National Institutes of Health Consensus Development Panel. NCI Monogr 1990;(9):3–8.

30. Hancock PJ, Epstein JB, Sadler GR. Oral and dental management related to radiation therapy for head and neck cancer. J Can Dent Assoc 2003;69(9):585–90.

31. Carl W. Local radiation and systemic chemotherapy: preventing and managing the oral complications. J Am Dent Assoc 1993;124(3):119–23.

32. Sennhenn-Kirchner S, Freund F, Grundmann S, et al. Dental therapy before and after radiotherapy–an evaluation on patients with head and neck malignancies. Clin Oral Investig 2009;13(2):157–64.

33. Omolehinwa TT, Akintoye SO. Chemical and radiation-associated jaw lesions. Dent Clin North Am 2016;60(1):265–77.

34. Damek-Poprawa M, Both S, Wright AC, et al. Onset of mandible and tibia osteoradionecrosis: a comparative pilot study in the rat. Oral Surg Oral Med Oral Pathol Oral Radiol 2013;115(2):201–11.

35. O'Dell K, Sinha U. Osteoradionecrosis. Oral Maxillofac Surg Clin North Am 2011; 23(3):455–64.

36. Fischer DJ, Epstein JB. Management of patients who have undergone head and neck cancer therapy. Dent Clin North Am 2008;52(1):39–60, viii.

37. Shaw RJ, Butterworth C. Hyperbaric oxygen in the management of late radiation injury to the head and neck. Part II: prevention. Br J Oral Maxillofac Surg 2011; 49(1):9–13.

38. Vissink A, Jansma J, Spijkervet FK, et al. Oral sequelae of head and neck radiotherapy. Crit Rev Oral Biol Med 2003;14(3):199–212.

39. Bardet E, Martin L, Calais G, et al. Subcutaneous compared with intravenous administration of amifostine in patients with head and neck cancer receiving radiotherapy: final results of the GORTEC2000-02 phase III randomized trial. J Clin Oncol 2011;29(2):127–33.

40. Chambers MS, Posner M, Jones CU, et al. Cevimeline for the treatment of postirradiation xerostomia in patients with head and neck cancer. Int J Radiat Oncol Biol Phys 2007;68(4):1102–9.

41. Atkinson JC, Grisius M, Massey W. Salivary hypofunction and xerostomia: diagnosis and treatment. Dent Clin North Am 2005;49(2):309–26.

42. Garcia MK, Chiang JS, Cohen L, et al. Acupuncture for radiation-induced xerostomia in patients with cancer: a pilot study. Head Neck 2009;31(10):1360–8.

43. Bensadoun RJ, Riesenbeck D, Lockhart PB, et al. A systematic review of trismus induced by cancer therapies in head and neck cancer patients. Support Care Cancer 2010;18(8):1033–8.

44. Dijkstra PU, Sterken MW, Pater R, et al. Exercise therapy for trismus in head and neck cancer. Oral Oncol 2007;43(4):389–94.

45. Scherpenhuizen A, van Waes AM, Janssen LM, et al. The effect of exercise ther-apy in head and neck cancer patients in the treatment of radiotherapy-induced trismus: a systematic review. Oral Oncol 2015;51(8):745–50.

46. Clark GT. The management of oromandibular motor disorders and facial spasms with injections of botulinum toxin. Phys Med Rehabil Clin N Am 2003;14(4): 727–48.

47. Epstein JB, Barasch A. Taste disorders in cancer patients: pathogenesis, and approach to assessment and management. Oral Oncol 2010;46(2):77–81.

48. Mosel DD, Bauer RL, Lynch DP, et al. Oral complications in the treatment of cancer patients. Oral Dis 2011;17(6):550–9.

49. Mossman K, Shatzman A, Chencharick J. Long-term effects of radiotherapy on taste and salivary function in man. Int J Radiat Oncol Biol Phys 1982;8(6):991–7.

50. Fernando IN, Patel T, Billingham L, et al. The effect of head and neck irradiation on taste dysfunction: a prospective study. Clin Oncol 1995;7(3):173–8.

51. Persohn E, Canta A, Schoepfer S, et al. Morphological and morphometric anal-ysis of paclitaxel and docetaxel-induced peripheral neuropathy in rats. Eur J Cancer 2005;41(10):1460–6.

52. Komaki R, Meyers CA, Shin DM, et al. Evaluation of cognitive function in patients with limited small cell lung cancer prior to and shortly following prophylactic cranial irradiation. Int J Radiat Oncol Biol Phys 1995;33(1):179–82.

53. Logan RM. Advances in understanding of toxicities of treatment for head and neck cancer. Oral Oncol 2009;45(10):844–8.

54. Clark GT, Ram S. Orofacial pain and neurosensory disorders and dysfunction in cancer patients. Dent Clin North Am 2008;52(1):183–202, ix-x.

55. de Leon-Casasola OA. Current developments in opioid therapy for management of cancer pain. Clin J pain 2008;24(Suppl 10):S3–7.

56. Jann MW, Slade JH. Antidepressant agents for the treatment of chronic pain and depression. Pharmacotherapy 2007;27(11):1571–87.

57. Mao J, Chen LL. Systemic lidocaine for neuropathic pain relief. Pain 2000;87(1): 7–17.

58. Pace A, Savarese A, Picardo M, et al. Neuroprotective effect of vitamin E supple-mentation in patients treated with cisplatin chemotherapy. J Clin Oncol 2003; 21(5):927–31.

59. Gedlicka C, Kornek GV, Schmid K, et al. Amelioration of docetaxel/cisplatin induced polyneuropathy by alpha-lipoic acid. Ann Oncol 2003;14(2):339–40.

60. Akintoye SO, Brennan MT, Graber CJ, et al. A retrospective investigation of advanced periodontal disease as a risk factor for septicemia in hematopoietic stem cell and bone marrow transplant recipients. Oral Surg Oral Med Oral Pathol Oral Radiol Endod 2002;94(5):581–8.

61. Lee MK, Nalliah RP, Kim MK, et al. Prevalence and impact of complications on outcomes in patients hospitalized for oral and oropharyngeal cancer treatment. Oral Surg Oral Med Oral Pathol Oral Radiol Endod 2011;112(5):581–91.

Impact of Oral Cancer on Quality of Life

Jesus Amadeo Valdez, DDS, MAS, Michael T. Brennan, DDS, MHS*

KEYWORDS

- Oral cancer • Quality of life • Psychosocial impact • Physical impact
- Financial impact

KEY POINTS

- Quality of life is an abstract, subjective, and multidimensional conceptualization of a patient's perception of self.
- The clinical manifestations of oral cancer and effects of treatment can lead to negative effects on the quality of life of the patient.
- Treatment of oral cancer has adverse effects on esthetics, speech, voice, and swallowing.
- Oral cancer treatment might require surgery that may result in altered facial appearance, which can cause social isolation and psychological distress.
- Treatment costs, work absences, medication prices, and other miscellaneous expenses can severely burden patients with oral cancer, especially patients with limited financial resources.

ORAL CANCER AND QUALITY OF LIFE

Quality of life is an abstract, subjective, and multidimensional concept that entails patient's self-perception in society. The World Health Organization defines quality of life as an individual's perception of his or her position in life in the context of the culture and value systems in which the patient lives and in relation to his or her goals, expectations, standards, and concerns.[1]

The clinical manifestations of oral cancer and effects of treatment can lead to negative effects on the quality of life of the patient. Patients may experience significant dysfunction in talking, swallowing, with alteration of cosmetic appearance, and sensory impairment, as well as chronic pain. All these factors when compounded lead to poor mental health.[2–5]

Disclosure Statement: We have no relationship with any commercial company that has direct financial interest in the subject matter or material discussed in this article.
Department of Oral Medicine, Carolinas Healthcare System, Carolinas Medical Center, PO Box 32861, Charlotte, NC 28232, USA
* Corresponding author.
E-mail address: mike.brennan@carolinashealthcare.org

QUALITY OF LIFE INSTRUMENTS

Substantial effort has been made to create cancer-specific instruments to measure quality of life (**Table 1**). These questionnaires or instruments are intended to reflect the difference between one's perceived reality and one's expectation or wishes.[6] Measuring these variances requires a complex health evaluation that includes physical, functional, physiologic, social, and spiritual domains. Some of the instruments focus on a specific symptom or functional aspect of the patient, and others are more global quality of life tools.[7]

The University of Washington Quality of Life Questionnaire is among the most frequent tools used to assess quality of life. A composite score is determined by adding together 9 domains and dividing by 9 to give a scale from 0 (for poor health) to 100 (good health). The 9 specific areas related to patients with head and neck cancer are pain, appearance, activity, recreation-entertainment, employment, speech, chewing, swallowing, and shoulder disability.[8]

The European Organization for Research and Treatment of Cancer Quality of Life Questionnaire aims to measure patients' health-related quality of life in oncology clinical trials, other well-designed research studies, and clinical practice. This instrument is specific to the type of cancer. This questionnaire consists of 35 questions about the symptoms and side effects of treatment. Eighteen questions address symptoms such as pain, swallowing, taste, and appearance. The next 12 questions measure functions such as eating, talking, social contact, and sexuality. Five more items are binary questions concerning analgesia, supplemental feeding, and weight.[9]

Table 1
Quality of life instruments

	UW-QOL	EORTC QLQ-H&N35	Liverpool Oral Rehabilitation
Number of Questions	15	35	25
Scale	Likert (5 point)	Likert (4 point)	Likert (4 point)
Scoring	• Range from 0 to 100. • Composite score is calculated by taking the averaging each domain score.	• Range from 1 to 4. • Composite score is a linear transformation of the sum of individual item scores	• Range from 1 to 4 • Composite score is the simple mean of individual item scores
Measures	• Pain • Appearance • Activity • Recreation • Swallowing • Chewing • Speech • Shoulder Involvement • Taste • Saliva • Mood • Anxiety • Overall QOL	• Pain • Swallowing • Senses • Speech • Social Eating • Social Contact • Sexuality	• Chewing • Swallowing • Oral Dryness • Speech • Drooling • Appearance • Social Life • Food Choice • Denture Issues

Abbreviations: EORTC, European Organization for Research and Treatment of Cancer.
Data from Refs.[8–10]

The Liverpool Oral Rehabilitation Questionnaire contains 25 items about oral function and denture satisfaction. The first 12 items assess general issues related to oral function and the remaining 13 items deal about dentures or denture satisfaction. Each item is rated on a 1 to 4 Likert scale ranging from never (1) to always (4).[10]

These examples of quality of life measures may be used in a clinical setting to evaluate for areas of need in patient management. Oral cancer has many physical, psychosocial, and financial implications, all of which can have large effects on the patients' quality of life.[4,5] Awareness of these impacts and their complexity can be used by health care providers to ensure patient access to information and resources.[6]

PHYSICAL IMPACT

Treatment of oral cancer has adverse effects on the face, speech, voice, and swallowing. Impairments can be attributed to the effects of the tumor itself or procedures before or during cancer treatment such as tracheostomy, pain from mucositis, xerostomia, amputation of oral structures, or fibrosis due to radiation treatment.[11] Some of these impairments can present before treatment is initiated, some are most troublesome during and immediately after treatment, and some can persist and worsen for years after treatment. Self-esteem can be affected when normal facial appearance or communication ability is altered by oral cancer treatment.[12]

Esthetics Impact

Oral cancer treatment may include surgery that involves removing large areas of facial features. Altered facial appearance can cause social isolation and psychological distress. Reconstructive surgery may be necessary to help the patient recover facial features and functions. Bone or tissue may be harvested from other body sites to replace lost tissue, including the labial mucosa, tongue, palate, or mandible. A maxillofacial prosthodontist can often fabricate dental and facial prostheses to diminish the effects of the surgical resection (**Figs. 1** and **2**).[13,14]

Speech Impact

Speech is usually affected by chemotherapy and radiation therapy. Typically, the severity is mild to moderate and is related primarily to treatment of the tongue, teeth, palate, and lips. Patients with oral cancer may have trouble articulating speech rapidly

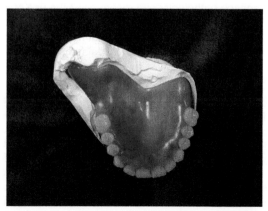

Fig. 1. Maxillary obturator. (*Courtesy of* Dr Robert Schortz, Carolinas HealthCare System, Charlotte, NC.)

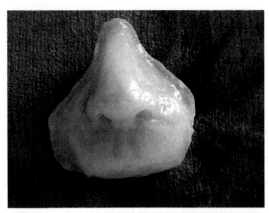

Fig. 2. Prosthesis used for restoring anatomy after a partial or complete removal of the nose. (*Courtesy of* Dr Robert Schortz, Carolinas HealthCare System, Charlotte, NC.)

when experiencing symptoms such as dry mouth or pain due to mucositis.[15] A speech pathologist must evaluate the patient before, during, and after cancer treatment. The goal is to return the patient to the highest satisfactory function in the shortest amount of time. Some speech problems may not require any intervention and simply resolve over time. More complex situations require therapy that depends on the severity of the issues. Treatment of these conditions can include muscle-strengthening exercises, controlled breathing, and management of nervousness when talking.[14]

Voice Impact

Voice quality in patients with oral cancer can be severely affected by different factors, including (1) impairment of vocal fold mobility, (2) altered tongue anatomy, and (3) chronic laryngeal edema. As a result, the patient's voice can become strained, wheezy, or harsh.[16] Patients with xerostomia may experience voice changes resulting from dryness of the laryngeal mucosa. Resonance can be altered when patients undergo changes in the palatal anatomy or edema in the oropharynx.[17] Speech pathologists are an important resource to patients with these conditions. They can instruct the patient on modified voice rest exercises during treatment and, if the patient has a tracheostomy, the speech pathologist can recommend the use of a 1-way speaking valve and provide training in its use. For hypernasality, a nose clip can be beneficial. The maxillofacial prosthodontist and speech pathologist collaborate closely for long-term management of patients with voice impairments.[14]

Swallowing Impact

Dysphagia is a common result of oral cancer treatment. Swallowing is directly affected by the inability to properly masticate due to mandibular resection, dental extractions, impairment of the mobility of the tongue, or scarring of the labial mucosa.[18] Patients with oral cancer have a higher risk of aspirating while eating due to the impact on efficiency and safety of swallowing. Swallowing function can also be affected years after radiation therapy. Tissue fibrosis ultimately can produce some degree of dysfunction.[19] To improve swallowing, a specialist may teach the patient different postures (head turn or chin tuck), maneuvers (breath hold before swallow), diet modifications (thickened fluids), or tongue exercises (tongue retraction). Alcohol abuse withdrawal syndrome can result in behaviors such as anxiety, irritability, and decreased cognition, which can alter the success of the swallowing interventions provided by the speech pathologist. In patients with extensive surgical involvement, an intraoral prosthetic appliance can have be a major improvement on the efficiency or safety or the oropharyngeal swallow. These prosthetics are designed individually, usually by a maxillofacial prosthodontist and a speech-language pathologist.[13,14]

PSYCHOSOCIAL IMPACT

Oral cancer represents a psychosocial challenge not only for patients but also for their family and diagnosing provider (**Fig. 3**). Not all patients are affected to the same degree; therefore, it is fundamental to have a complete understanding of the range of psychological and social obstacles patients may experience.[20–25] Government institutions, nonprofit organizations, and internet forums are some of the available resources to assist patients with attaining balance in their lives at diagnosis, during treatment, and through survivorship.[21]

Impact on the Patient

The diagnosis of oral cancer often evokes a shock reaction in the patient and, often, they will seek an explanation to amend feelings of guilt for falling ill to this disease.[23] Usually, patients with cancer will experience progressive fears, such as fear of the unknown; death anxiety; fear of loneliness; fear of change; fear of loss of control; fear of regression; and, particularly, the fear of loss of identity.[22] The patient may approach these fears with an array of varying defense measures that they may use either constructively or destructively during the course of their disease.[13,21]

The most common defense measure used by patients with cancer is denial. Denial is an unconscious defense that prevents the patient from acknowledging an unpleasant reality.[26] Denial can be manifested through different approaches, including intellectualizations, humor, and anger. This coping technique can also affect pathologic

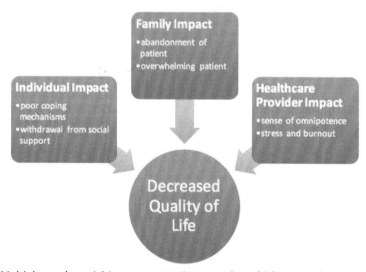

Fig. 3. Multiple psychosocial impacts on patient's quality of life. (*Data from* Schnaper N, Kellner TK. Psychosocial effect of cancer on the patient and the family. In: Peterson DE, Elias EG, Sonis ST, editors. Head and neck management of the cancer patient. Boston: Martinus Nijhoff Publishing; 1986. p. 503–7.)

processes when it interferes with disease treatment. For example, a patient in denial may see a mass on his face but readily defer treatment, believing that there is no need for intervention. In these cases, denial is used in a destructive manner, diminishing chances for successful treatment and rehabilitation. However, this mechanism has the potential to be used constructively by permitting patients with oral cancer to have hope for a cure or a better future without acknowledging detrimental aspects of the disease.[13,14]

Projection is a coping mechanism by which the patient with oral cancer attributes a false feeling to another person. An example of this is in the case in which a patient believes their health care provider is hurting them and does not intend to cure them for their own benefit. This point of view can cause stress in the patient and difficulty in the patient–provider relationship. A poor patient–provider relationship can lead to poor outcomes for the patient due to provider frustration or patient noncompliance.[13]

Another mechanism of defense is repression, or unconscious forgetting, and its variations, which include suppression (conscious forgetting), regression (reversion to an early life stage), and magical thinking (expecting health care professionals to be omnipotent and assure a cure for their disease). Repression can lead to false judgments surrounding the patient's course of treatment or disease prognosis.[25]

Patient personality and individuality is an important consideration in management of patients with oral cancer. The individual whose premorbid personality was flexible, aggressive, and embodied a sense of self-worth and humor may view their disease as a hurdle or challenge to overcome.[22] They will likely be more compliant during treatment, participate in activities they enjoy, and seek social support. However, patients lacking these premorbid personality traits may be more likely to revert to unhelpful coping and defense mechanisms, potentially making their treatment more complicated and compromising posttreatment outcomes. It is important to recognize that each patient, has a unique personality and will cope in their own way with their own assets or liabilities.[24]

For the most part, treatment of patients with oral cancer involves surgical intervention. This experience, or anticipation of this experience, can provoke emotional trauma and can seem to the patient as a life-or-death threat. The patient reaction to surgery is complex and fluctuates based on their personality, defense systems, and accumulated fears and traumas. Distortions of the face typically play a significant role in any surgical experience due to the threat of change in one's physical appearance or body image.[26] In many social situations, patients with facial scarring or facial disfigurement are approached with negativity. This stigmatized response (horror, fear, or revulsion), or the patients' expectation of this response may cause further emotional stress in surgical oral cancer cases.[14,21]

In the postoperative stage of treatment, the patient may believe that their body image, and on a larger scale, their sense of identity, is shattered. They may believe that an obvious facial misconfiguration, such as a tongue or jaw resection, will cause them to be rejected or unwelcome in their social circles.[27] After surgery, these patients may experience social withdrawal, depression, rage, and impotency, with some even regressing to infantile behavior.[28]

Some postoperative patients will develop a hyperawareness of their disfigurement, causing them to anticipate social stigmatization and even wear scarves or surgical masks to prevent drawing the attention of others.[29] Patients may develop frustration in efforts to communicate with others because facial expression and speech are important to communication and social success but may be limited by their disfigurement. Patients in these situations may show apathy, bitterness, and quibbling toward society. This leads to the experience of social death, by which the patient withdraws from all forms of social interaction and support.[25]

In addition to cancer therapy, a comprehensive rehabilitation, including plastic surgery, dental prostheses, psychotherapy, and occupational and physical therapy, may help the patient revert from the negative effects of cancer treatment.[29] This may include rebuilding feelings of self-worth, increasing physical functionality, and reestablishing lost social support.[14] Group therapy with other survivors can also be a useful support mechanism, although individual therapy is often preferred by patients with facial involvement.[26] Psychological treatment should be implemented into standard of care practice for patients with oral cancer. Psychiatric medications may also be helpful to provide comfort for the patient during a difficult disease course. In this case, referral to a psychotherapist is useful to ensure comprehensive patient care.[13]

Impact on the Family

Family is a fundamental component in the journey of a patient with oral cancer. The family's reactions and emotions regarding the patient's disease may either have a positive or negative effect on the patient as they move through the stages of diagnosis, treatment, and rehabilitation, and should be considered in the patient's plan of care.[25] There are many directions from which families may approach their loved one's disease. Some may emotionally overwhelm the patient, whereas others may opt to abandon the patient at the time of the diagnosis. Balanced support from the patient's family is important and neither extreme is positive in regard to patient outcomes.[30]

In many cases, the family's most immediate problem is the threat of loss or separation from their loved-one, which can evoke sensations of sadness, sorrow, and anxiety. Usually, the family process of grief and mourning begins with shock and sense of unreality, followed by emotional releases; hostility; depression; physical symptoms (anorexia, guilt, panic); and, finally, the experience of readjustment to reality.[31] Families, like individuals, have different personalities, characteristics, and dynamics. All of these phases, with different intensities, may be encountered from the families of patients with oral cancer.[24,25,30]

More intense reactions can begin pathologic processes in family members experiencing grief. These reactions include delayed grief, chronic grief, overdependence, reckless and dangerous behavior, and even physical illness. These reactions require the intervention of specialists and need to be identified early by psychotherapists.[27,32]

A controversial aspect that has a direct effect on the family and society is the matter of whether a patient's behavior makes them cancer-prone.[32] This theory suggests that emotional states function etiologically and implies that patient's sins contribute to patient's condition. The idea that the patient's alcoholism, use of tobacco, or lack of ambition are causative in the development of oral cancer is reinforced in the minds of others based on the observation of lower socioeconomic status, older age, or appearance.[13,14]

Support from family and friends in the patient's course of disease is incredibly important. The family or other social support group must be able to accept that the period of adjustment to disease diagnosis and treatment can be extensive and that affection must be steady.[33]

Impact on Health Care Providers

Health care providers are a source of knowledge and support to the patient with oral cancer. However, health care providers are also human with their own personality and virtues. Some providers find it impossible to work with patients with oral cancer, others may find it difficult, and others may establish a comfortable clinical distance and even experience gratification in the field.[14,34]

The sense of omnipotence in a health care provider can cause poor judgment and negatively affect the patient.[26] At this point, the provider is concerned more about curing the patient than caring for them and any setback on the part of the patient is experienced as a failure of omnipotence.[35] This is unconscious in many health care providers but manifests itself in subtle ways such as anger toward the patient, avoidance, or patronization, which can significantly impact the relationship between the patient and their health care provider.[14,36]

When it becomes evident that a patient may have poor outcomes or a terminal prognosis, the omnipotent provider is compelled by guilt and accountability to abandon the patient before death, thus avoiding retribution.[26] Health care providers who have chosen to work in the cancer field should be emotionally mature and have a clear appreciation for their sense of omnipotence.[14,35,37]

Health care providers are vulnerable individuals and can be subject to exhaustion from the stress of their profession. Attentiveness to signs of depression is fundamental; self-medication, excessive alcohol intake, and fatigue are indicators of burnout.[38] Patients and health care providers must create a relationship of trust to provide the basis to tolerate the desolation associated with the oral cancer diagnosis.[39]

FINANCIAL IMPACT

A large percentage of patients receiving oral cancer treatment reported their condition has a significant impact on their finances and that the cost of the treatment was a major burden to their family members.[40]

Treatment costs, work absences, medication prices and other miscellaneous expenses can severely burden patients with oral cancer, especially patients with limited financial resources.[41]

Financial struggle can cause significant stress in patients undergoing oral cancer treatment. The complex financial issues associated with cancer diagnosis within the family are often hidden from friends and health care professionals as the family struggles to make decisions, manage emotions, and preserve the family unit.[42]

Patients may be hesitant to request financial aid. It is incumbent on the team of health care providers to support their patients by connecting them to community resources that can provide assistance with financial management of disease. Social workers, case managers, and nurse navigators are often knowledgeable in these areas and can provide information on insurance coverage for patients and connecting with local and national nonprofits for monetary assistance.[14]

A referral to social workers and financial advisors may be appropriate for patients who have financial burdens as a result of their oral cancer diagnoses. A significant percentage of patients may need financial counseling to budget expected and unexpected oral cancer costs.[40]

Employment for oral cancer survivors represents safety, self-esteem, and quality of life. However, patients may not always return to work after rehabilitation due to different reasons. Patients may encounter several physical challenges to the oral cavity that may influence patient employability and ability to maintain a job. Anxiety, xerostomia, trismus, sticky saliva, teeth pain, and problems with social eating and social contacts can distress the patient's ability to function with the work environment.[43]

One study reported that patients with oral cancer who were employed at the time of the diagnosis discontinued work due to 5 significant factors: (1) fatigue, (2) change in speech, (3) change in eating, (4) pain or discomfort, and (5) change in appearance.[44] A separate study reported that the way in which patients handle unemployment can affect overall adjustment during the course of their condition.[45] Factors such as physical health, financial resources, and patient personality will contribute to the unemployment adjustment. Individuals with higher self-esteem, perceived control, and higher levels of optimism are more likely to cope successfully.[26] Patients with physical implications may develop depression or anxiety and may struggle more in regard to unemployment. This type of patient may have poor outcomes in other psychosocial areas and be at risk for engaging in high-risk behaviors such as substance abuse.[13]

Family counseling is advantageous in certain situations. Unemployment of the patient will often cause role changes within the family structure, leaving another family member responsible for the lost income. This can cause stress within the family and feelings of guilt in the patient.[46] The patient's accessibility to financial support can also affect the patient's capacity to follow through on a referral for therapy or counseling. For patients who cannot afford to pay for treatment or psychotherapy on their own, access to community resources can lessen their anxiety when these services are advised.[42]

SUMMARY

Quality of life considerations are important in evaluating treatment outcomes of oral cancer. The diagnosis of oral cancer itself can have implications on the patient's perspective of their experience, which can alter the trajectory of treatment and rehabilitation, creating more long-term effects. Several aspects of a patient's life, including psychosocial, physical, and financial, are all affected by the various stages of oral cancer and play a part in contributing to negative or positive effects in the patient's quality of life. Health care providers should be attentive not only to the clinical effects of treatment but also to quality of life issues because it will improve overall patient care and satisfaction.

REFERENCES

1. The World Health Organization Quality of Life Group. The World Health Organization Quality of Life assessment (WHOQOL): position paper from the World Health Organization. Soc Sci Med 1995;41:1403–9.
2. Abendstein H, Nordgren M, Boysen M, et al. Quality of life and head and neck cancer: a 5 year prospective study. Laryngoscope 2005;115:2183–92.
3. Oskam IM, Verdonck-de Leeuw IM, Aaronson NK, et al. Prospective evaluation of health-related quality of life in long-term oral and oropharyngeal cancer survivors and the perceived need for supportive care. Oral Oncol 2013;49:443–8.
4. Hilarius DL, Kloeg PH, Gundy CM, et al. Use of health-related quality-of-life assessments in daily clinical oncology nursing practice: a community hospital-based intervention study. Cancer 2008;113:628–37.
5. Crombie AK, Farah CS, Batstone MD. Health-related quality of life of patients treated with primary chemoradiotherapy for oral cavity squamous cell carcinoma: a comparison with surgery. Br J Oral Maxillofac Surg 2014;52:111–7.
6. Tadakamadla J, Kumar S, Lallo R, et al. Development and validation of a quality-of-life questionnaire for patients with oral potentially malignant disorders. Oral Surg Oral Med Oral Pathol Oral Radiol 2017;123:338–49.
7. Gupta B, Kumar N, Johnson NW, et al. Predictors affecting quality of life in patients with upper aerodigestive tract cancers: a case-control study from India. Oral Surg Oral Med Oral Pathol Oral Radiol 2017;123:550–8.

8. Hassan SJ, Weymuller EA. Assessment of quality of life in head and neck cancer patients. Head Neck 1993;15:485–96.

9. Aaronson N, Ahmedzai S, Bergman B, et al. The European Organization for Research and Treatment of Cancer QLQ-C30: a quality-of-life instrument for use in international clinical trials in oncology. J Natl Cancer Inst 1993;85(5): 365–75.

10. Pace-Balzan A, Cawood JI, Howell R, et al. The Liverpool Oral Rehabilitation Questionnaire: a pilot study. J Oral Rehabil 2004;31(6):609–17.

11. So WK, Chan RJ, Chan DN, et al. Quality-of-life among head and neck cancer survivors at one year after treatment a systematic review. Eur J Cancer 2012; 48:2391–408.

12. Chen SC, Huang BS, Lin CY. Depression and predictors in Taiwanese survivors with oral cancer. Asian Pac J Cancer Prev 2013;14:4571–6.

13. Collins SL. Controversies in multimodality therapy for head and neck cancer: clinical and biologic perspectives. In: Thawley SE, Panje WR, Batsakis MD, et al, editors. Comprehensive management of head and neck tumors. Philadelphia: W.B. Saunders Co; 1999. p. 251–5.

14. Schroeder E, Witt ME. Psychosocial Challenges. In: Hass ML, McBride DL, editors. Managing the oral effects of cancer treatment: diagnosis to survivorship. Philadelphia: Oncology Nursing Society; 2011. p. 205–18.

15. Funk GF, Karnell LH, Christensen AJ. Long-term health-related quality of life in survivors of head and neck cancer. Arch Otolaryngol Head Neck Surg 2012; 138:123–33.

16. Cooper JS, Fu K, Marks J, et al. Late effects of radiation therapy in the head and neck region. Int J Radiat Oncol Biol Phys 1995;31:1141–64.

17. Scrimger R, Kanji A, Parliament M, et al. Correlation between saliva production and quality of life measurement in head and neck cancer patients treated with intensity-modulated radiotherapy. Am J Clin Oncol 2007;30:271–7.

18. Payakachat N, Ounpraseuth S, Suen JY. Late complications and long-term quality of life for survivors (>5 years) with history of head and neck cancer. Head Neck 2013;35:819–25.

19. Kovacs AF, Stefenelli U, Thorn G. Long-term quality of life after intensified multimodality treatment of oral cancer including intra-arterial induction chemotherapy and adjuvant chemoradiation. Ann Maxillofac Surg 2015;5:26–31.

20. Thomas L, Moore EJ, Olsen KD, et al. Long-term quality of life in young adults treated for oral cavity squamous cell cancer. Ann Otol Rhinol Laryngol 2012; 121:395–401.

21. Reich M, Leemans CR, Vermorken JB, et al. Best practices in the management of the psycho-oncologic aspects of head and neck cancer patients: recommendations from the European Head and Neck Cancer Society make sense campaign. Ann Oncol 2014;25:2115–24.

22. Rapoport Y, Kreitler S, Chaitchik S, et al. Psychosocial problems in head-and-neck cancer patients and their change with time since diagnosis. Ann Oncol 1993;4:69–73.

23. Singer S, Krauss O, Keszte J, et al. Predictors of emotional distress in patients with head and neck cancer. Head Neck 2012;34:180–7.

24. Hammerlid E, Mercke C, Sullivan M, et al. A prospective quality of life study of patients with laryngeal carcinoma by tumor stage and different radiation therapy schedules. Laryngoscope 1998;108:747–59.

25. Zwahlen RA, Dannemann C, Gratz KW, et al. Quality of life and psychiatric morbidity in patients successfully treated for oral cavity squamous cell cancer and their wives. J Oral Maxillofac Surg 2008;66:1125–32.
26. Schnaper N, Kellner TK. Phychosocial effect of cancer on the patient and the family. In: Peterson DE, Elias EG, Sonis ST, editors. Head and neck management of the cancer patient. Boston: Martinus Nijhoff Publishing; 1986. p. 503–7.
27. Howren MB, Christensen AJ, Karnell LH, et al. Psychological factors associated with head and neck cancer treatment and survivorship: evidence and opportunities for behavioral medicine. J Consult Clin Psychol 2013;81(2):299–317.
28. De Boer MF, Van Den Borne B, Pruyn JF, et al. Psychosocial and physical correlates of survival and recurrence in patients with head and neck carcinoma: results of a 6-year longitudinal study. Cancer 1998;83:2567–79.
29. Mehanna HM, De Boer MF, Morton RP. The association of psycho-social factors and survival in head and neck cancer. Clin Otolaryngol 2008;33:83–9.
30. Shu-Ching C, Mei-Chu T, Chih-Lien L, et al. Support needs of patients with oral cancer and burden to their family caregivers. Cancer Nurs 2009;32:473–81.
31. Semple CJ, Sullivan K, Dunwoody L, et al. Psychosocial interventions for patients with head and neck cancer: past, present, and future. Cancer Nurs 2004;27:434–44.
32. Riley JL, Dodd VJ, Muller KE, et al. Psychosocial factors associated with mouth and throat cancer examinations in rural Florida. Am J Public Health 2012;102(2):e7–14.
33. Rodríguez VM, Corona R, Bodurtha JN, et al. Family ties: the role of family context in family health history communication about cancer. J Health Commun 2016;21(3):346–55.
34. Meier DE, Back AL, Morrison RS. The inner life of physicians and the care of the seriously ill. JAMA 2001;286(23):3007–14.
35. Ramirez AJ, Graham J, Richards MA, et al. Burnout and psychiatric disorder among cancer clinicians. Br J Cancer 1995;71(6):1263–9.
36. Kash KM, Holland JC, Breitbart W, et al. Stress and burnout in oncology. Oncology (Williston Park) 2000;14(11):1621–33.
37. Linzer M, Visser MR, Oort FJ, et al. Predicting and preventing physician burnout: results from the United States and the Netherlands. Am J Med 2001;111(2):170–5.
38. Kash KM, Holland JC. Special problems of physicians and house staff in oncology. In: Holland JC, Rowland JH, editors. Handbook of psychooncology. New York: Oxford University Press; 1989. p. 647–57.
39. Jones G, Sagar S, Wong R. The effects of stress on oncology staff. CMAJ 2000;163(7):807.
40. USA Today, Kaiser Family Foundation, Harvard School of Public Health. National Survey of Households Affected by Cancer. http://www.kff.org/health-costs/poll-finding/usa-todaykaiser-familyfoundationharvard-school-of-public-2/. November 2006. Accessed July 7, 2017.
41. Yabroff KR, Dowling EC, Guy GP, et al. Financial hardship associated with cancer in the United States: findings from a population-based sample of adult cancer survivors. J Clin Oncol 2016;34(3):259–67.
42. Kent EE, Forsythe LP, Yabroff KR, et al. Are survivors who report cancer-related financial problems more likely to forgo or delay medical care? Cancer 2013;119(20):3710–7.
43. Verdonck-de Leeuw IM, van Bleek WJ, Leemans CR, et al. Employment and return to work in head and neck cancer survivors. Oral Oncol 2009;46(1):56–60.

44. Buckwalter AE, Karnell LH, Smith RB, et al. Patient-reported factors associated with discontinuing employment following head and neck cancer treatment. Arch Otolaryngol Head Neck Surg 2007;133(5):464–70.
45. McKee-Ryan F, Song Z, Wanberg CR, et al. Psychological and Physical well-being during unemployment: a meta-analytic study. J Appl Psychol 2005;90(1): 53–76.
46. Yabroff KR, Lund J, Kepka D, et al. Economic burden of cancer in the US: estimates, projections, and future research. Cancer Epidemiol Biomarkers Prev 2011;20(10):2006–14.

Moving?

Make sure your subscription moves with you!

To notify us of your new address, find your **Clinics Account Number** (located on your mailing label above your name), and contact customer service at:

Email: journalscustomerservice-usa@elsevier.com

800-654-2452 (subscribers in the U.S. & Canada)
314-447-8871 (subscribers outside of the U.S. & Canada)

Fax number: 314-447-8029

Elsevier Health Sciences Division
Subscription Customer Service
3251 Riverport Lane
Maryland Heights, MO 63043

*To ensure uninterrupted delivery of your subscription, please notify us at least 4 weeks in advance of move.

Printed and bound by CPI Group (UK) Ltd, Croydon, CR0 4YY

03/10/2024

01040395-0016